W9-CMK-160

Ending Neglect

The Elimination of Tuberculosis in the United States

Lawrence Geiter, *Editor*

Committee on the Elimination of Tuberculosis
in the United States

Division of Health Promotion and
Disease Prevention

INSTITUTE OF MEDICINE

NATIONAL ACADEMY PRESS
Washington, D.C.

NATIONAL ACADEMY PRESS • 2101 Constitution Avenue, N.W. • Washington, DC 20418

NOTICE: The project that is the subject of this report was approved by the Governing Board of the National Research Council, whose members are drawn from the councils of the National Academy of Sciences, the National Academy of Engineering, and the Institute of Medicine. The members of the committee responsible for the report were chosen for their special competences and with regard for appropriate balance.

This project has been funded entirely with federal funds from the Centers for Disease Control and Prevention, under Contract No. 200-98-0012. The views presented are those of the Institute of Medicine Committee on the Elimination of Tuberculosis in the United States and are not necessarily those of the funding organization.

Library of Congress Cataloging-in-Publication Data

Institute of Medicine (U.S.). Committee on the Elimination of Tuberculosis in
    the United States. Ending neglect : the elimination of tuberculosis in the
    United States / Lawrence Geiter, editor; Committee on the Elimination of
    Tuberculosis in the United States, Division of Health Promotion and
    Disease Prevention, Institute of Medicine.
      p. ; cm.
    Includes bibliographical references and index.
    ISBN 0-309-07028-7
      1. Tuberculosis—United States. I. Geiter, Lawrence. II. Title.
    [DNLM: 1. Tuberculosis, Pulmonary—prevention & control—United States
    WF 300 I59e 2000]
    RC313.A2 I55 2000
    614.5′42′0973—dc21

                                            00-056115

The full text of this report is available on line at **www.nap.edu.**

For more information about the Institute of Medicine, visit the IOM home page at **www.iom.edu.**

Printed in the United States of America

The serpent has been a symbol of long life, healing, and knowledge among almost all cultures and religions since the beginning of recorded history. The image adopted as a logotype by the Institute of Medicine is based on a relief carving from ancient Greece, now held by the Staatliche Museen in Berlin.

Cover: Modigliani. Self-portrait, 1919. Oil on canvas. Museu de Arte Contemporanea da Universidade de Sao Paulo. Collection M and Madame Francisco-Matarazzo Sabrinho.

"Knowing is not enough; we must apply.
Willing is not enough; we must do."
—Goethe

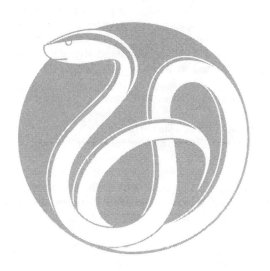

INSTITUTE OF MEDICINE

Shaping the Future for Health

THE NATIONAL ACADEMIES

National Academy of Sciences
National Academy of Engineering
Institute of Medicine
National Research Council

The **National Academy of Sciences** is a private, nonprofit, self-perpetuating society of distinguished scholars engaged in scientific and engineering research, dedicated to the furtherance of science and technology and to their use for the general welfare. Upon the authority of the charter granted to it by the Congress in 1863, the Academy has a mandate that requires it to advise the federal government on scientific and technical matters. Dr. Bruce M. Alberts is president of the National Academy of Sciences.

The **National Academy of Engineering** was established in 1964, under the charter of the National Academy of Sciences, as a parallel organization of outstanding engineers. It is autonomous in its administration and in the selection of its members, sharing with the National Academy of Sciences the responsibility for advising the federal government. The National Academy of Engineering also sponsors engineering programs aimed at meeting national needs, encourages education and research, and recognizes the superior achievements of engineers. Dr. William A. Wulf is president of the National Academy of Engineering.

The **Institute of Medicine** was established in 1970 by the National Academy of Sciences to secure the services of eminent members of appropriate professions in the examination of policy matters pertaining to the health of the public. The Institute acts under the responsibility given to the National Academy of Sciences by its congressional charter to be an adviser to the federal government and, upon its own initiative, to identify issues of medical care, research, and education. Dr. Kenneth I. Shine is president of the Institute of Medicine.

The **National Research Council** was organized by the National Academy of Sciences in 1916 to associate the broad community of science and technology with the Academy's purposes of furthering knowledge and advising the federal government. Functioning in accordance with general policies determined by the Academy, the Council has become the principal operating agency of both the National Academy of Sciences and the National Academy of Engineering in providing services to the government, the public, and the scientific and engineering communities. The Council is administered jointly by both Academies and the Institute of Medicine. Dr. Bruce M. Alberts and Dr. William A. Wulf are chairman and vice chairman, respectively, of the National Research Council.

COMMITTEE ON THE ELIMINATION OF TUBERCULOSIS IN THE UNITED STATES

---

*Resigned in June 1999 for personal reasons unrelated to committee activities.

v

Preface

In 1905, in his book *The Life of Reason*, the poet and philosopher George Santayana wrote "Those who do not remember the past are condemned to repeat it." This statement is particularly apropos now as we attempt to develop a plan for the future elimination of tuberculosis in the United States, ever mindful of the lessons that can be gleaned from the historical record.

The incidence of tuberculosis in this country and in Europe began to decline in the late 19th and early 20th centuries with improving social and economic conditions. By the 1930s, the possibility of eliminating this leading infectious cause of death globally began to be pondered by public health experts. The introduction in the early 1950s of the first effective antimicrobial drugs for treatment of tuberculosis was followed in the 1960s by the closing of many tuberculosis hospitals and sanatoriums. The elimination of this dread disease seemed feasible at that time provided public interest and government expenditures commensurate with the task could be marshaled and sustained. This was not to be the case; rather, the declining incidence of tuberculosis in the United States induced complacency and neglect for this disease. Indeed, after several years of decreasing federal support, in 1972 categorical federal funding for tuberculosis control was eliminated entirely. It was not reinstated for 9 years, and then only at a very reduced level. In addition, the scientific community and funding agencies largely disregarded tuberculosis, deeming it of insufficient importance to warrant a high research priority. As a consequence of this lack of funding and research interest, scientific publications in this field decreased by almost 50 percent between 1968 and 1980. The price of this neglect has been the resurgence of tuberculosis in the United States in the late 1980s and early 1990s, with major costs in suffering, death, and economic losses. Reversal of the ensuing increased case rates, many involving patients whose infecting microorganisms were multidrug resistant, was accomplished only with great difficulty and required energetic tuberculosis control measures and markedly increased public expenditures.

We are now at a critical juncture. On the one hand, control of tuberculosis in the United States has been regained and we are at an all-time low in the number of new cases (18,361 in 1998). On the other hand, we are particularly vulnerable again to the complacency and neglect that comes with declining numbers of cases. Now is the time to commit to the abolition of the recurrent cycles of neglect followed by resurgence that have been the history of tuberculosis in the latter half of the past century.

In 1989, almost simultaneous with an unexpected upsurge in the incidence of tuberculosis in the United States, the Centers for Disease Control and Prevention (CDC) and the Advisory Council for the Elimination of Tuberculosis (ACET) developed a strategic national plan to reduce the incidence of tuberculosis to 3.5 cases per 100,000 persons by the year 2000, and by 2010, to less than 1 case per 1 million population. However, in place of the steady (about 7 percent per year) decline of cases prior to 1985, between 1985 and 1992 cases of tuberculosis increased from 22,210 to 26,673 per year. Since the latter date, the incidence of tuberculosis in the United States has resumed its former rate of decline (again about 7 percent annually) to 18,361 cases in 1998, or 6.8 cases per 100,000 population. At this rate of decline it would take 60 more years to reach the stated 1989 CDC/ACET goal for 2010 (1 case per 1 million population) unless changes were made in the methods used for the control of tuberculosis.

This Institute of Medicine report, *Ending Neglect: The Elimination of Tuberculosis in the United States,* undertaken under sponsorship from the CDC, reviews the lessons learned from the neglect of tuberculosis between the late 1960s and the early 1990s and reaffirms committing to the goal of eliminating tuberculosis in the United States, defined as a case rate of less than 1 case per 1 million population per year. Clearly, to meet this goal aggressive and decisive actions beyond what is now in effect will be required. The report details the following recommendations in full, but a few are listed here:

• **Maintaining control of tuberculosis while adjusting control measures to declining incidence of disease and changing systems of health care management.** This will be integral to interrupting transmission of tuberculosis and, most important, to preventing the emergence of multidrug-resistant tuberculosis. Among measures to ensure this, all states should mandate completion of therapy for all patients with active tuberculosis. In addition, to advance toward elimination of tuberculosis in areas of the country with already low rates of tuberculosis, activities toward elimination should be regionalized through both federal and multistate initiatives to improve access to and more efficient utilization of clinical, epidemiological, case management, and laboratory services. Federal categorical funding for tuberculosis control should be retained, providing dedicated resources for this purpose while allowing maximum flexibility and efficiency in its implementation.

• **Accelerating the rate of decline of tuberculosis (aimed at elimination) by increasing efforts at targeted tuberculin testing and treatment of latent infection.** This would involve development of more effective methodologies to identify persons with recently acquired tuberculosis infection and increased efforts to evaluate and treat latent infection in persons at high risk of subsequent progression to active disease. Tuberculin skin testing should be required in the medical evaluation of immigrants applying for visas from countries with high rates of tuberculosis. Those found to be tuberculin positive should be required to undergo an evaluation for tuberculosis, and, when appropriate, complete an approved course of treatment for latent infection before receiving their permanent residency card. Similar tuberculin testing should be required of all inmates of correctional institutions and, when indicated, completion of an appropriate course of treatment. Programs of targeted tuberculin skin testing and treatment of latent infection should be intensified for other high-incidence populations such as homeless individuals, undocumented immigrants, and intravenous drug abusers, as indicated by local epidemiological considerations.

• **Developing new tools necessary for the ultimate elimination of tuberculosis, including new diagnostic tests for latent infection, new treatments and an effective vaccine.**

• **Increasing involvement of the United States in global tuberculosis control, recognizing the fact that tuberculosis is not constrained by national boundaries and that increasing proportions of new cases in this country are developing in individuals born in countries with high incidences of tuberculosis.**

• **Mobilizing and sustaining public support and commitment for elimination of tuberculosis and regularly measuring progress toward that goal.**

This committee comprised 13 individuals with expertise in tuberculosis (clinical aspects, epidemiology, mycobacteriological research, prevention and control, and health education), ethics, public health policy and infectious disease eradication, state correctional health services, international health and general infectious disease. In response to public comment on committee composition that noted an absence of experts on public health tuberculosis laboratories, a special report on this subject was commissioned and is included in this report (Appendix D). The committee met five times, and these included public sessions at four of the meetings. In particular, the final public session was held to provide for full and open discussion on issues raised regarding tuberculin testing (and prophylactic therapy when appropriate) of immigrants to the United States from countries with high incidence rates of tuberculosis. This discussion benefited from the involvement of experts in ethics, immigration law, and public policy as well as representatives from the Immigration and Naturalization Service, CDC, and the Department of State.

In addition, committee members conducted site visits to a variety of sites (state and local health departments, CDC, public hospitals, homeless facilities, and facilities for nonadherent infectious patients placed under legal orders to complete therapy), selected to represent a full range of the problems and issues in current tuberculosis control. These sites included ones in Atlanta, San Diego, Seattle/King County and Tacoma/Pierce County in Washington, Boston, Washington, D.C., and Augusta and Portland in Maine (Appendix C).

The report is organized in the following fashion. Chapter 1 covers the fundamentals of tuberculosis, including its transmission, pathogenesis, diagnosis, treatment, and control. Chapter 2 reviews the history of tuberculosis in the United States, analyzes the implications of disease elimination, and discusses the ethical issues in moving toward elimination. Chapter 3 considers many of the challenges of tuberculosis programs to prevent a resurgence of tuberculosis in this country as the number of cases declines: maintaining high skill levels and quality of care, needs for performance standards, developing necessary information systems for evaluating case management and disease control, and the increasing use of managed care and the potential for regionalization of control and diagnostic efforts. Chapter 4 makes the case for accelerating the rate of decline of tuberculosis through use of targeted tuberculin skin testing programs and treatment of latent infection; improving methodologies for contact tracing, examination and treatment; changing the medical examination of visa applicants from high-incidence countries to include tuberculin testing and treatment, where appropriate, in those that are tuberculin positive. This change from established procedure evoked the most discussion and greatest attention from the committee. The approaches discussed in this chapter should speed up the current rate of decline of tuberculosis and advance the eventual elimination of this disease in the United States. Chapter 5 describes the current status of tuberculosis research and pinpoints the research needs, both short term (newer methodologies for the diagnosis and treatment of latent tuberculosis) and longer term (vaccine development), that need to be fulfilled to make the elimination of tuberculosis a reality. Chapter 6 identifies the need for an enhanced role of the United States in global tuberculosis control, both from the point of view of self-interest and humanitarian considerations. Chapter 7 covers the important role of public advocacy efforts to develop and sustain the political commitment needed to make elimination of tuberculosis a reality.

The committee would like to thank the numerous experts from various governmental agencies, academic institutions, professional organizations, and groups working with immigrants, migrant workers, and the homeless who made presentations at its meetings, thus ensuring consideration of a broad set of views in the development of its recommendations (Appendix B). The committee is particularly grateful to Lawrence Geiter, Ph.D., the IOM study director, for his untiring efforts in working our discussions and contributions into a coherent, thorough, and well-reasoned report within a year of our first meeting, with the assistance of his staff, Donna Almario, Elizabeth Epstein, and Patricia Spaulding. We wish to thank Robert Fullilove, Ed.D., liaison to the IOM Board on Health Promotion and Disease Prevention, who attended and participated in our meetings and discussions, and George Comstock, Dr.P.H., who was originally a committee member until forced to withdraw because of an illness in his family. We also wish to thank Kenneth I. Shine, M.D., president of IOM; Kathleen Stratton, acting director of the Division of Health Promotion and Disease Prevention; and Rose Martinez, director of the Division of Health Promotion and Disease Prevention, for their support and insights.

Morton N. Swartz, M.D., *Chair*

Acknowledgments

The committee wishes to express its appreciation to the many individuals who contributed to the completion of this project. We especially want to thank our consultant, Robert C. Good, Ph.D., whose paper appears as Appendix D, and the many workshop presenters who provided the committee with a wealth of information (see Appendix B).

This report has been reviewed in draft form by individuals chosen for their diverse perspectives and technical expertise, in accordance with procedures approved by the NRC's Report Review Committee. The purpose of this independent review is to provide candid and critical comments that will assist the institution in making the published report as sound as possible and to ensure that the report meets institutional standards for objectivity, evidence, and responsiveness to the study charge. The review comments and draft manuscript remain confidential to protect the integrity of the deliberative process.

We wish to thank the following individuals for their participation in the review of this report:

Mary Ellen Avery, Harvard Medical School
Mark Barnes, Proskauer Rose LLP, New York City
Jerrold Ellner, New Jersey Medical School, University of Medicine and Dentistry of New Jersey
Lee B. Reichman, New Jersey Medical School National Tuberculosis Center, Newark
Barbara G. Rosenkrantz, Harvard University

Sarah Royce, Tuberculosis Control Branch, California Department of
Health Services, Berkeley
Steven Schroeder, The Robert Wood Johnson Foundation, Princeton,
New Jersey
Zena Stein, Gertude H. Sergievsky Center, Columbia University

While the individuals listed above have provided constructive comments and suggestions, it must be emphasized that responsibility for the final content of this report rests entirely with the authoring committee and the institution.

Contents

Ending Neglect

Executive Summary

Institute of Medicine Study on the Elimination of
Tuberculosis in the United States

STATEMENT OF TASK

The study will review the current state of tuberculosis mortality,
morbidity, and prevention/control efforts in the United States, with
special emphasis on regional and other variations; assess special
challenges and solutions for the high proportion of U.S. cases of
TB [tuberculosis] in foreign-born persons; and review the current
state of research and development in the United States on new
diagnostics and therapeutics for TB prevention, control, and elimination; review the extent of multidrug-resistant tuberculosis and
analyze factors that contribute to its development; and examine
the role of the United States in international efforts at tuberculosis
control. The committee will develop conclusions and recommendations regarding: a framework to guide a national campaign to
eliminate TB in the United States; region-specific action steps required to work towards that goal; research needs and priorities for
national TB elimination; information for health care providers and
the public regarding the importance of vigilant and continued attention to TB control; health plan (fee-for-service and managed
care) responsibilities for TB prevention and control; federal, state,
and local public health policy maker's responsibilities and options
regarding infrastructure needs; and strategies for U.S. contributions to worldwide TB prevention and control, leading to worldwide
TB elimination.

Tuberculosis, an infectious disease caused by *Mycobacterium tuberculosis*, has plagued humanity since before recorded history and, globally, is still the leading infectious cause of death. As social and economic conditions began to improve in Europe and North America in the late 19th century, tuberculosis rates began to decline in the late 1800s and early 1900s and in the 1930s public health experts began to speculate about the possibility of elimination of this dread disease. Later, with the discovery of antimicrobial agents effective for the treatment of tuberculosis, the elimination of the disease seemed achievable. Plans for tuberculosis elimination were advanced, first to take advantage of the closing of no-longer-needed tuberculosis hospitals and sanatoriums to fund an aggressive drive against tuberculosis in the 1960s and then to take advantage of the retreat of tuberculosis into focal pockets in the United States and strive for elimination in the 1980s. None of these calls for elimination was heeded, and, to the contrary, categorical federal funding for tuberculosis was eliminated in 1972.

The price of the neglect reflected in the funding reductions was a resurgence of tuberculosis throughout the United States. This increase in tuberculosis incidence was greatest in places where the tuberculosis and human immunodeficiency virus epidemics overlapped and where new immigrants from countries with high rates of tuberculosis tended to settle. However, without question the major reason for the resurgence of tuberculosis was the deterioration of the public health infrastructure essential for the control of tuberculosis. It has been estimated that the monetary costs of losing control of tuberculosis were in excess of $1 billion in New York City alone. Not only was the increase in the number of cases of tuberculosis great concern, but also of rising concern was the specter of multidrug-resistant tuberculosis, a form of the disease that requires treatment with less effective, toxic, and expensive drugs and that is often fatal.

In the past 6 to 7 years the decline in number of cases of tuberculosis has resumed, and all-time lows in both the number and incidence of cases have been achieved, clearly a laudable achievement. The question now confronting the United States is whether another cycle of neglect will be allowed to begin or whether, instead, decisive action will be taken to eliminate the disease. At a minimum, strategies for tuberculosis control will have to adapt to a declining incidence and the changing health care environment. For example, the private sector is becoming increasingly involved in both tuberculosis treatment and tuberculosis prevention, which will require effective programs of training and education for private sector clinicians, patients, and targeted segments of the general public. The increasing reliance on managed care will require changes in approaches to tuberculosis treatment but will also offer opportunities to ensure quality of care through effective contracts and clinical standards. Health departments will need to develop approaches to integrating tuberculosis control with other public health programs while maintaining the capacity and focus to ensure program effectiveness.

The changes outlined above will enable a continuation of the decline in the number and rates of tuberculosis; however, because they fall well short of the goal of elimination, the nation will continue to be susceptible to another resurgence when interest inevitably wanes or perturbations in epidemiological circumstances occur. To begin advancing toward the elimination of tuberculosis, aggressive new efforts must be implemented to identify those who are at the greatest risk of disease through targeted programs of tuberculin skin testing coupled with treatment for latent tuberculosis infection. The highest priority is the identification and treatment of infected contacts of individuals with infectious cases of active tuberculosis. In many parts of the country foreign-born individuals from countries with high rates of tuberculosis also make up a high-priority group; however, because the epidemiology of the disease varies from place to place within the United States, other high-risk groups must be identified locally. Prevention of tuberculosis in foreign-born immigrants from countries with high rates of tuberculosis presents a challenge. The proportion of U.S. cases among individuals in this group is steadily increasing, and soon more than half of all cases of tuberculosis in the United States will be among foreign-born individuals. To address the disease among some foreign-born individuals with tuberculosis, those applying for immigrant visas could be required to undergo tuberculin skin testing as part of the medical examination already required for immigrants to the United States and could be required to complete examination and treatment for tuberculosis or latent tuberculosis infection (when indicated) before receiving documents for permanent U.S. residency. This takes advantage of procedures already required at the time of immigration and identifies individuals during their period of highest risk for tuberculosis, the immigrant's first 5 years in the United States.

Unquestionably, such a policy will be difficult to implement. New resources will be required for health departments to review or conduct medical examinations for newly arrived immigrants and to ensure that treatment is appropriately prescribed and supervised. The Centers for Disease Control and Prevention (CDC) and the Immigration and Naturalization Service (INS) will also require new resources to provide the training and quality assurance necessary to conduct the overseas screening and to ensure the efficient flow of information to health departments. Approaches to implementation of this program should proceed in a stepwise fashion through a series of pilot studies, with each demonstrating effective implementation procedures. Despite the recognized difficulty, an analysis of the effect of this approach demonstrates that it is likely to have a substantial impact on the decline in the rate of tuberculosis in the United States. Not only will screening and treatment of foreign-born individuals target an epidemiologically important group in the United States, but it also will develop and promote the infrastructure needed for aggressive programs of prevention for other high-risk populations already in the United States.

However, even these efforts will not lead to the elimination of tuberculosis. Elimination of tuberculosis will require continued research and the development of new tools. The past decade has seen increased resources for tuberculosis research. Recently, the complete genome of *M. tuberculosis* has been sequenced, providing a wealth of information and setting the stage for truly meaningful and important advances in tuberculosis prevention, diagnosis, and treatment. Globally, the focus has been on the development of a vaccine. However, for the United States the greater needs are for better tests for the diagnosis of latent tuberculosis infection and the identification of individuals who are at the greatest risk of developing active tuberculosis. Advances such as these, together with more effective treatment of latent infection, will lead to the elimination of tuberculosis in the United States.

Elimination of tuberculosis in the United States will also require that the global pandemic of tuberculosis be addressed effectively. As noted earlier, tuberculosis is a leading cause of death worldwide, even though it is a readily treatable and preventable disease. Moreover, the World Bank has identified treatment of tuberculosis as highly cost-effective. The United States must increase its engagement in the global effort to control tuberculosis through participation in multilateral efforts, such as the Stop TB Initiative, and through bilateral initiatives with countries where the rates of tuberculosis are high and that present special circumstances, such as Mexico, which shares a large land border with the United States.

The key to achieving tuberculosis elimination will be through social mobilization and maintaining the public interest and commitment necessary to provide sufficient resources for the effort. The tendency to shift attention and resources away from the elimination of tuberculosis will increase as the number of cases decreases. Only an aggressive effort aimed at building political commitment can prevent the elimination of funding for tuberculosis research and before the elimination of the disease, leading to yet another period of neglect.

The committee agrees with the current policy, advocated by the Advisory Council for the Elimination of Tuberculosis, of committing to the goal of eliminating tuberculosis in the United States, defined as a case rate of less than 1 per 1 million population per year. This plan was updated in a 10-year review published by the Council in 1999 in the *Morbidity and Mortality Weekly Report* (MMWR) and this report supports their conclusions.

The magnitude of this task is clear. Even if intensified tuberculosis control efforts increase the annual rate of decline from the current 7.5 percent to a 10 percent rate of decline for the next 10 years new tools are developed during that time and those new tools result in a doubling of the annual rate of decline to 20 percent thereafter, it will still take until 2035 to reach the target for tuberculosis elimination. To achieve the goal of tuberculosis elimination in the United States the committee recommends steps that fall into five main categories:

1. Maintaining control of tuberculosis while adapting to a declining incidence of disease and changing systems of health care financing and management.
2. Speeding the decline of tuberculosis and advance toward the elimination of tuberculosis through increased efforts related to targeted tuberculin skin testing and treatment of latent infection.
3. Developing the tools needed for the ultimate elimination of tuberculosis, new diagnostic tests, particularly for diagnosis of infection, new treatments, and an effective vaccine.
4. Increasing U.S. engagement in global efforts to control elimination.
5. Mobilizing support for elimination and regularly measuring progress toward that goal.

MAINTAINING CONTROL

The control of tuberculosis requires the ability to identify and cure individuals with active tuberculosis. The current decline in the number of cases and rates of tuberculosis would indicate that most jurisdictions in the United States are achieving this objective, usually by using a patient-centered approach to therapy and ensuring that patients complete treatment. However, as the numbers of cases decline it will become increasingly difficult to maintain expertise in tuberculosis control and provide a focus within the public health system for the surveillance and management of infectious individuals. These challenges, however, are occurring at the same time that systems of health care financing are changing, including an increasing reliance on managed care organizations and private providers for the delivery of medical services. Those with tuberculosis are eligible for Medicaid, and many health departments are taking advantage of this to fund a variety of services, including directly observed therapy. In addition, tuberculin skin testing and treatment of latent infection are eligible for Medicaid reimbursement. Medicaid, Medicare, and other insurance plans could be important sources of funds for expanded tuberculosis prevention programs. An important aspect of Medicaid funding is that, as an entitlement, the funding provided grows with the number of patients served and is theoretically unlimited.

The loss of categorical funding for tuberculosis was a major factor in the decline in the tuberculosis control infrastructure and the subsequent resurgence of tuberculosis in the 1980s and 1990s. Categorical funding will ensure that support for tuberculosis control is not neglected again and can also be justified on the basis of the fact that tuberculosis is a serious, infectious disease spread through casual contact and requires a national approach for its control. However, as the number of cases declines, increased integration of tuberculosis with other public health activities will be required in some areas. Bureaucratic obstacles to shared resources (e.g., use of cofunding for personnel or facilities with funds from multiple programs) need to be identified and eliminated to allow the more efficient use of financial and other resources. It is also important to maintain funding to maintain activities at their current levels. Level funding for tuberculosis control programs can result in de facto cuts in funding because of the high rates of inflation associated with medical services and can put the current decline in the numbers of cases at risk.

(Note: The first digit in the recommendation number refers to the chapter in the report that contains the recommendation and supporting information.)

Recommendation 3.1 To permanently interrupt the transmission of tuberculosis and prevent the emergence of multidrug-resistant tuberculosis, the committee recommends that

  • **All states have health regulations that mandate completion of therapy (treatment to cure) for all patients with active tuberculosis.**
  • **All treatment be administered in the context of patient-centered programs that are based on individual patient characteristics. Such programs must be the standard of care for patients with tuberculosis in all settings.**

Recommendation 3.2 To ensure the most efficient application of existing resources, the committee recommends that

  • **New program standards be developed and used by CDC and state and local health departments to evaluate program performance.**
  • **Standardized, flexible case management systems be developed to provide the information needed for the evaluation measurements. These systems should be integrated with existing case management systems and other automated public health data systems whenever possible.**

Recommendation 3.3 To make further progress toward the elimination of tuberculosis in regions of the country experiencing low rates of disease, the committee recommends that

• Tuberculosis elimination activities be regionalized through a combination of federal and multistate initiatives to provide better access to and more efficient utilization of clinical, epidemiological, and other technical services.
• Protocols and action plans be developed jointly by CDC and the states for use by state and local health departments to enable planning for the availability of adequate resources.
• State and local health departments develop case management plans to ensure a uniform high quality of care for patients with tuberculosis and tuberculosis infection in their jurisdictions.

Recommendation 3.4 To maintain quality in tuberculosis care and control services in an era of increased use of managed care systems and privatization of services, the committee recommends that

• When it is determined that tuberculosis diagnosis and treatment services can be provided more efficiently outside of the public health department, the delivery of such services be governed by well-designed contracts that specify performance measures and responsibilities.
• Federal categorical funding for tuberculosis control be retained. Funding at the local level should provide sufficient dedicated resources for tuberculosis control but should be structured to provide maximum flexibility and efficiency.
• Both public and private health insurance programs be billed for tuberculosis diagnostic and treatment services whenever possible but tuberculosis services should never be denied due to a patient's inability to make a co-payment.

Recommendation 3.5 To promote a well-trained medical (in a broad sense) workforce and educated public, the committee recommends that

• The Strategic Plan for Tuberculosis Training and Education, which contains the blueprint that addresses the training and educational needs for tuberculosis control, be fully funded.
• Programs for the education of patients with tuberculosis be developed and funded.
• Funding be provided for government, academic, and nongovernmental agencies to work in collaboration with international partners to develop training and educational materials.

SPEEDING THE DECLINE

After ensuring the control of tuberculosis through the provision of adequate treatment of individuals with active tuberculosis, the second priority is targeted tuberculin skin testing and treatment of latent infection, which includes the identification and treatment of contacts. This measure serves to protect the health of the individual and will accelerate the decline in tuberculosis case rates. Previously, tuberculosis was believed to be largely transmitted through prolonged, close exposure, such as in the household. Recent experience has demonstrated, however, that there are many instances of *M. tuberculosis* transmission occurring outside the household, in a variety of environments. Therefore, the search for persons newly infected with *M. tuberculosis* (contact investigation) must be broadened.

The proportion of new tuberculosis cases in the United States among foreign-born individuals has been steadily increasing. The period of greatest risk of tuberculosis for individuals who immigrate to the United States from countries with high rates of tuberculosis is during their first 5 years in this country. Recent guidelines from CDC have emphasized the importance of identifying immigrants from high-incidence countries as soon as possible after their arrival in the United States and providing them with tuberculin skin testing and treatment for latent infection, when indicated. The addition of tuberculin skin testing to the medical evaluation for immigrant visa applicants from countries with high rates of tuberculosis and linking of evaluation and treatment for tuberculosis to receipt of permanent residency status could facilitate this process. The committee discussed this recommendation at great length and recognizes that this will entail a difficult and complicated process and will require significant additional resources for state and local health departments, CDC, and INS. Such a program may need to be implemented in a stepwise fashion, by using pilot programs that focus on the highest-risk populations, upgrading the capacities of local health departments and CDC and INS systems, and carefully evaluating the results. In addition, it will be important to collect data concerning the safety among recent immigrant populations of the new short-course regimens that may be the preferred treatment. The extraordinarily high risk of tuberculosis in newly arrived immigrants from high-incidence countries justifies this effort.

The majority of inmates of correctional facilities have demographic characteristics that put them at higher risk of having tuberculosis infection. The importance of preventing cases of tuberculosis in correctional facilities is magnified by the ease with which new infections can be transmitted, should an infectious case of tuberculosis occur in the close setting of a jail or prison.

Increased testing and treatment for contacts, newly arrived immigrants, and inmates of correctional facilities will have significant impacts but there will still be high-risk populations who must be identified locally. These include groups such as HIV-infected individuals, homeless people, intravenous drug abusers, and undocumented immigrants. Successful programs for targeted testing and treatment of latent infection have been designed for these populations and many involve close collaboration with the community-based organizations, neighborhood health centers, and private providers that already provide medical care to these individuals.

Recommendation 4.1 To limit the spread of tuberculosis from infectious patients to their contacts, the committee recommends that more effective methodologies for the identification of persons with recently acquired tuberculosis infection, especially persons exposed to patients with new cases of tuberculosis, be developed and efforts be increased to evaluate appropriately and treat latent infection in all persons who meet the criteria for treatment for such infections.

Recommendation 4.2 To prevent the development of tuberculosis among individuals with latent tuberculosis infection, the committee recommends that

• **Tuberculin skin testing be required as part of the medical evaluation for immigrant visa applicants from countries with high rates of tuberculosis, a Class B4 immigration waiver designation be created for persons with normal chest radiographs and positive tuberculin skin tests, and all tuberculin-positive Class B immigrants be required to undergo an evaluation for tuberculosis and, when indicated, complete an approved course of treatment for latent infection before receiving a permanent residency card ("green card"). Implementation should be in a stepwise fashion and pilot programs should evaluate strategies and assess costs.**

• **Tuberculin testing be required of all inmates of correctional facilities and completion of an approved course of treatment, when indicated, be required, with referral to the appropriate public health agency for all inmates released before completion of treatment.**

• **Programs of targeted tuberculin skin testing and treatment of latent infection be increased for high-incidence groups, such as HIV-infected individuals, undocumented immigrants, homeless individuals, and intravenous drug abusers, as determined by local epidemiological circumstances.**

DEVELOPING NEW TOOLS

Tuberculosis elimination is not possible with the tools that are available currently. Fortunately, an investment in the development of a tuberculosis research infrastructure and expertise during the past 7 years has the research community poised for progress in the development of new tools and strategies. The first priority area for research is development of an understanding of latent infection. The ability to identify individuals who are truly infected with *M. tuberculosis* and who are at risk for disease will tremendously simplify the process of tuberculosis elimination in the United States. An important area of research that has been lacking is behavioral and social science research targeted toward understanding and improving patient adherence with therapy. This is an increasingly complex and troublesome question as the characteristics of tuberculosis patients change and become ever more varied. The committee estimates that the National Institutes of Health (NIH), CDC, the U.S. Food and Drug Administration, and the U.S. Agency for International Development annual research budgets for tuberculosis will have to be increased to approximately $280 million (approximately tripled). Moreover, industry and private foundations must substantially increase their investments in basic and applied research to achieve the recommendations presented above. To enable the most efficient use of the increased funds, the increase should be phased in and then maintained over a significant time period.

Recommendation 5.1 To advance the development of tuberculosis vaccines, the committee recommends that the plans outlined in the *Blueprint for Tuberculosis Vaccine Development*, published by NIH in 1998, be fully implemented.

Recommendation 5.2 To advance the development of diagnostic tests and new drugs for both latent infection and active disease, action plans should be developed and implemented. CDC should then exploit its expertise in population-based research to evaluate and define the role of promising products.

Recommendation 5.3 To promote better understanding of patient and provider nonadherence with tuberculosis treatment recommendations and guidelines, a plan for a behavioral and social science research agenda should be developed and implemented.

Recommendation 5.4 To encourage private-sector product development, the global market for tuberculosis diagnostic tests, drugs,

and vaccines should be better characterized and access to these markets for these new products should be facilitated.

Recommendation 5.5 To define the applicability of any new tools to the international arena and facilitate their development, the U.S. Agency for International Development (AID), NIH, and CDC should build upon international relationships and expertise to conduct research.

ENGAGING IN GLOBAL TUBERCULOSIS CONTROL

Tuberculosis is a leading cause of death worldwide, even though it is a readily treatable and preventable disease. Although an altruistic argument for promoting the global control of tuberculosis can easily be advanced, worldwide control of this disease is also in the nation's self-interest. The proportion of foreign-born patients with tuberculosis in the United States has been steadily increasing. In 1998, 41 percent of all patients with tuberculosis were foreign-born. It benefits the United States to help strengthen tuberculosis control programs globally, particularly in the countries that are the sources of the most tuberculosis cases imported into the United States. Tuberculosis will not be eliminated in the United States until the worldwide pandemic is brought under control.

Recommendation 6.1 To decrease the number of foreign-born individuals with tuberculosis in the United States, to minimize the spread and impact of multidrug-resistant tuberculosis, and to improve global health, the committee recommends that

• The United States expand and strengthen its role in global tuberculosis control efforts, contributing to these efforts in a substantial manner through bilateral and multilateral international efforts.

• The United States contribute to global tuberculosis control efforts through targeted use of financial, technical, and human resources and research, all guided by a carefully considered strategic plan.

• The United States work in close coordination with other government and international agencies. In particular, the United States should continue its active role in and support of the Stop TB Initiative.

• AID, CDC, and NIH should jointly develop and publish strategic plans to guide U.S. involvement in global tuberculosis control efforts.

MOBILIZING SUPPORT FOR ELIMINATION

The United States has a long history of social mobilization efforts in support of tuberculosis control. Social mobilization provides for the enlistment and coordination of efforts by myriad groups and individuals. Advocacy to influence policy makers and education of patients, health care providers, and the general public are critical activities.

An ad hoc World Health Organization committee identified the lack of political will on the part of national governments as a fundamental constraint to developing and sustaining effective tuberculosis control programs. Social mobilization is necessary to build and sustain political will in the United States and can lead to similar efforts internationally.

Recommendation 7.1 To build public support and sustain public interest and commitment to the elimination of tuberculosis, the committee recommends that CDC significantly increase resources for activities to secure and sustain public understanding and support for tuberculosis elimination efforts at the national, state, and local levels, including programs to increase knowledge among targeted groups of the general public.

Recommendation 7.2 To increase the effectiveness of mobilization efforts the committee recommends that the National Coalition for the Elimination of Tuberculosis continue to provide leadership and oversight and that CDC continue to work in collaboration with the coalition to secure the support and participation of nontraditional public health partners, ensure the development of state and local coalitions, and evaluate public understanding and support for tuberculosis elimination efforts with the assistance of public opinion research experts.

Recommendation 7.3 To assess the impacts of these recommendations and to measure progress toward accomplishing the elimination of tuberculosis, the committee recommends that, 3 years after the publication of this report and periodically thereafter, the Office of the Secretary of Health and Human Services conduct an evaluation of the actions taken in response to the recommendations in this report.

1

Fundamentals of Tuberculosis and Tuberculosis Control

HISTORICAL EPIDEMIOLOGY

Tuberculosis has affected humans since before recorded history. Some speculate that the first cases may have been attributable to *Mycobacterium bovis* infections acquired by humans from domesticated animals and that *Mycobacterium tuberculosis* may have evolved from *M. bovis* (Daniel, 1994). Whatever the source, modeling of epidemiological data suggests that tuberculosis became endemic in human populations when stable social networks of about 200 to 440 people were established, about 10,000 years ago (McGrath, 1988). Tuberculosis is thought to have occurred in Europe, the Americas, and North Africa from prehistoric times. Mummies and skeletal remains that show evidence of deformities characteristic of spinal tuberculosis, with accompanying indications of fibrotic lesions in the lung, provide evidence of the disease in northern Africa as far back as 3,000 years ago (Morse et al., 1964). Similar evidence from remains in Peru (Salo et al., 1994) and Chile (Arriaza et al., 1995), supported by the presence of restriction fragment length polymorphism analysis (commonly referred to as "DNA fingerprinting") patterns that are characteristic of *M. tuberculosis*, indicates that tuberculosis was present in pre-Columbian times. However, tuberculosis does not seem to have been introduced into sub-Saharan Africa, East Asia, or the Pacific Islands until after contact with Europeans during the period of colonization.

Tuberculosis grew to epidemic proportions in Europe beginning in the early 1600s as populations shifted to expanding cities and population densities increased (Dubos and Dubos, 1952). Conditions were ideal for

13

of becoming active at any time, although the factors that govern reactivation are not known. Thus, individuals with a latent infection are at risk of developing active tuberculosis at any time in the future. The risk is greatest during the first 2 years after being infected, during which time about 5 percent of infected persons develop active tuberculosis. Another 5 percent of infected persons will develop active tuberculosis at a later time in their lives. It is generally thought that approximately 90 percent of individuals with latent infection will never develop tuberculosis (Comstock et al., 1974). If active tuberculosis develops in the lungs and becomes sufficiently advanced, tubercle bacilli will be expelled by any maneuver that produces rapid exhalation, such as coughing, sneezing, yelling, or singing. These bacilli can then cause new infections in susceptible individuals and perpetuate the cycle.

It is the airborne route by which tuberculosis infection is spread that causes the disease to be a public health threat. Individuals with untreated tuberculosis can unknowingly spread the infection to others in their environment. Generally, however, tuberculosis is not highly infectious and transmission usually requires close and prolonged exposure. Individuals living in the household of a person with active tuberculosis are usually at the highest risk of infection, but recent epidemiological investigations have shown that tuberculosis infection can be acquired in more casual settings (Curtis et al., 1999; Mangura et al., 1998; Tabet et al., 1994), such as a bar, a church, or a classroom. The degree of infectiousness of a person with tuberculosis can be inferred from the results of microscopic examination of sputum. Patients who are excreting sufficient numbers of bacilli that the bacilli can be seen on microscopic examination (i.e., the patient is smear positive) are more infectious than patients who are smear negative (Grzybowski and Allen, 1964; Shaw and Wynn-Williams, 1954). However, patients who are smear negative and culture positive can transmit the infection, and even those patients who have negative smears and cultures but who have radiographic evidence of tuberculosis. can infect others (Behr et al., 1999).

DIAGNOSIS AND TREATMENT

Active Tuberculosis

The signs and symptoms of tuberculosis depend on the sites involved. In general, however, systemic symptoms and signs, such as fatigue, anorexia, weight loss, and persistent low-grade fever, occur with any site of involvement. Respiratory tract symptoms, especially cough, predominate when the lungs are involved. Epidemiological circumstances and the presence of signs and symptoms associated with the disease suggest the diagnosis of tuberculosis. Pulmonary tuberculosis may be suggested by abnormalities on a chest radiograph. The finding of acid-fast organisms on microscopic examination of sputum or other material is more highly suggestive of the diagnosis. However, the "gold standard" for the diagnosis of tuberculosis is isolation of the tubercle bacillus in a culture of a patient's sputum or another biological specimen. In the United States, about 80 percent of reported cases of tuberculosis are confirmed by a positive culture. Other diagnostic tests, based on the amplification of nucleic acids (RNA and DNA) specific for *M. tuberculosis*, have been developed, but their exact role in diagnosis is still being defined.

The standard treatment for tuberculosis caused by drug-sensitive organisms is a 6-month regimen consisting of four drugs given for 2 months, followed by two drugs given for 4 months. The two most important drugs, given throughout the 6-month course of therapy, are isoniazid and rifampin. Although the regimen is relatively simple, its administration is quite complicated. Daily ingestion of the eight or nine pills often required during the first phase of therapy can be a daunting and confusing prospect. Even severely ill patients are often symptom-free within a few weeks, and nearly all appear to be cured within a few months. If the treatment is not continued to completion, however, the patient may experience a relapse, and the relapse rate for patients who do not continue treatment to completion is high. A variety of forms of patient-centered care are used to promote adherence with therapy. The most effective way of ensuring that patients are taking their medication is to use directly observed therapy, which involves having a member of the health care team observe the patient take each dose of each drug. Directly observed therapy can be provided in the clinic, the patient's residence, or any mutually agreed upon site. Nearly all patients who have tuberculosis caused by drug-sensitive organisms and who complete therapy will be cured, and the risk of relapse is very low.

Drug-resistant organisms result from random mutations in the tubercle bacilli, and drug-resistant disease results when an ineffective regimen is used or when an effective regimen is taken irregularly. The threat of drug resistance, and the threat of multiple-drug resistance in particular, is another aspect of tuberculosis that is causing it to be an increasing public health threat. Tuberculosis caused by isoniazid-resistant organisms is still readily treatable and may not require the addition of any new drugs to the regimen or an extension of therapy. Tuberculosis caused by rifampin-resistant organisms can also usually be cured, but the duration of therapy must be extended to twelve months or more. Tuberculosis caused by organisms resistant to both isoniazid and rifampin requires treatment with much more expensive and toxic drugs for periods of 24 months or more, and the disease may be incurable in some patients.

Latent Tuberculosis Infection

As noted earlier, latent tuberculosis infection occurs when, because of an effective immune response, the host halts the multiplication of tubercle bacilli but the organisms are not killed. Latent infection causes no symptoms and can be diagnosed only by a positive tuberculin skin test together with an evaluation that does not indicate the presence of active tuberculosis. The tuberculin skin test, however, has several inherent weaknesses. Although the test has a fairly high sensitivity (the proportion of truly infected persons who react to the test), some truly infected people will not have a positive reaction. This happens when the infection is very recent (a positive skin test develops 2 to 10 weeks after infection) or when the immune system is compromised (e.g., in individuals with human immunodeficiency virus [HIV] infection, certain malignancies and other disease states, or individuals who are taking immune-suppressive drugs). Of greater importance is the relatively poor specificity (the proportion of uninfected individuals who test negative) of the skin test. Persons infected with non-*M. tuberculosis* mycobacteria and those recently vaccinated with BCG (a vaccine against tuberculosis used in many countries outside the United States) will often have a positive reaction.

When the specificity of a test is less than 100 percent, false-positive results will occur; the lower the true prevalence of infection, the larger the proportion of positive results that are false positive becomes. In the United States the prevalence of true tuberculosis infection is believed to be less than 10 percent. Even with a 10 percent prevalence of infection, a tuberculin skin test with a 100 percent sensitivity and a 95 percent specificity would result in about one-third of all positive test results being falsely positive. This is why screening of the general population by a broad-based tuberculin skin test is impractical. However, in a population with a 35 percent prevalence of infection, a tuberculin skin test with 100 percent sensitivity and 95 percent specificity would produce false-positive results for less than 10 percent of samples tested; thus, tuberculin skin testing should be targeted to groups in which there is a high incidence of tuberculosis because it provides a more accurate result.

Treatment of persons with latent tuberculosis infection can greatly reduce the incidence of tuberculosis. A series of clinical trials has shown the effectiveness of isoniazid ranging from 92 percent in preventing active tuberculosis in patients when adherence is high, to 26 percent when adherence is low (Ferebee, 1970). A study of 3-, 6-, and 12-month regimens showed that a 12-month regimen was optimal but additional analysis indicates that a regimen of at least 9 months of treatment gives nearly as much protection as a regimen of 12 months (International Union Against Tuberculosis Committee on Prophylaxis, 1982).

Concerns about liver toxicity have limited the use of isoniazid for the treatment of latent infection. Thus, there has been controversy over the use of isoniazid in persons at relatively low risk of tuberculosis. In contrast, the use of isoniazid has never been challenged for individuals at a high risk of tuberculosis, including recent tuberculin skin test converters, contacts of individuals with infectious cases of tuberculosis, immigrants from countries with high rates of tuberculosis, and individuals with certain medical conditions, especially HIV infection. A recent report of a 7-year study of patients receiving isoniazid for treatment of latent infection showed a rate of clinical hepatitis of only 0.1 percent (11 cases in 11,141 patients), with no deaths and only one hospitalization (Nolan et al., 1999).

In addition to isoniazid, rifampin-based regimens have recently been recommended as treatment for latent tuberculosis infection. The current recommended regimens for treatment of latent infection include isoniazid for 9 months (with an option for isoniazid for 6 months), rifampin and pyrazinamide for 2 months, and rifampin alone for 4 months (American Thoracic Society and Centers for Disease Control and Prevention, 2000). Although the rifampin-pyrazinamide regimen has the obvious advantages of being much shorter, the experience with this regimen is relatively limited, a high rate of hepatotoxicity was observed in an early pilot study, and programs that use this regimen have been encouraged to maintain surveillance for adverse reactions to this regimen.

PRINCIPLES OF TUBERCULOSIS CONTROL

In the United States, public health departments are charged with the following responsibilities for tuberculosis control (Centers for Disease Control and Prevention, 1995; Etkind, 1993; Simone and Fujiwara, 1999). Ensuring that persons who are suspected of having active tuberculosis disease are identified as soon as possible, evaluated appropriately, placed on the recommended course of treatment, and complete therapy as prescribed is the prime responsibility of the health department. Mechanisms to accomplish this goal are numerous and varied given the diverse population groups affected by tuberculosis today. Ideally, they include patient-centered programs that assess each patient's needs and that identify a treatment plan to ensure the completion of therapy (Chaulk, 1999). The treatment plan may include the use of any or all of the following:

• Enablers (defined as "anything that helps the patient to more readily complete therapy" [American Lung Association of South Carolina and the Division of Tuberculosis Control, South Carolina Department of Health and Environmental Control, 1989]). These may include transportation vouchers, assistance with child care, or the use of extended clinic hours.

- Incentives (defined as "something which will motivate the patient to take his medicine, keep clinic appointments or do anything else that is necessary to successfully carry out program goals" [Frieden et al., 1995]). These may include food stamps, coupons for fast-food restaurants, assistance with finding housing, etc. Incentives are tailored to meet the needs of the individual and, therefore, must be valued by that individual. This may vary considerably among patients as well as among communities.
- Alternate treatment delivery sites, such as workplaces, park benches, street corners, ferry and subway stations.
- Directly-observed therapy (where providers observe the patient ingesting the medication).
- Outreach workers whose responsibilities may include adherence monitoring, sputum collection, education, contact investigation assistance, social service assistance, translation, and so forth.
- Use of strategies that are specifically designed to overcome the social or cultural obstacles to treatment completion.

Treatment plans are developed in conjunction with the patient, the physician or nurse, a social worker (as necessary), and other team members, as appropriate. The plan is reviewed periodically and revised as needed through meetings between the patient and the assigned provider and often more formally through case and cohort reviews. The reviews must include the entire team providing care to the patient, including physicians, nurses, social workers, outreach workers, and so forth. A continuum of increasingly restrictive measures is used beginning with the use of the least restrictive measure (such as monthly monitoring in the outpatient setting) to the most restrictive measure (legally required hospitalization). These measures are invoked in a stepwise fashion to ensure that the needs and the rights of the patient are taken into account and the public's health is protected as well.

The second tuberculosis control priority is contact investigation and follow-up. Every individual with an infectious case or a suspected case of tuberculosis (index case) should prompt a thorough epidemiological investigation to identify other individuals who have potentially been exposed and who are therefore at high risk of having been infected by the index patient. These individuals should be evaluated for latent tuberculosis infection, and if they are found to have latent tuberculosis infection they should be placed on treatment and monitored until completion of therapy. Chapter 4 highlights the subject of contact investigations, their current use, and suggestions for improvement.

The final priority for health departments is the identification of persons who, because of epidemiological circumstances, are at high risk of having latent tuberculosis infection. This is done by:

- Analysis of local epidemiological data and targeting of high-incidence groups for specific screening projects.
- Ensuring that patients, once identified via screening programs, have access to appropriate and adequate tuberculosis services. This again is dependent on the high-risk group being targeted and may require services being provided outside of the "traditional tuberculosis clinic" system.
- Ensuring that patients are evaluated and placed on treatment for latent tuberculosis infection (as appropriate).
- Ensuring their completion of therapy. Screening without follow-up does not serve the needs of the patients or public health.

Health departments attain these goals by structuring their tuberculosis services within the framework of essential functions as described in the Institute of Medicine report, *The Future of Public Health* (Institute of Medicine 1988). This framework includes assessment (epidemiology and surveillance), policy development, and assurance (patient and contact management and education and training). The methods by which these goals are addressed vary according to morbidity rates, public health infrastructure capacity, and resources.

REFERENCES

American Lung Association of South Carolina and the Division of Tuberculosis Control, South Carolina Department of Health and Environmental Control. 1989. *Tuberculosis Control Enablers and Incentives.* Columbia: Author.

American Thoracic Society and Centers for Disease Control and Prevention. 2000. Targeted tuberculosis testing and treatment of latent infection. *Am J Respir Crit Care Med* 161:5221–5247.

Arriaza BT, Salo W, Aufderheide AC, and Holcomb TA. 1995. Pre-columbian tuberculosis in northern Chile: Molecular and skeletal evidence. *Am J Phys Anthropol* 98(1):37–45.

Behr MA, Warren SA, Salamon H, Hopewell PC, Ponce de Leon A, Daley CL, Small PM. 1999. Transmission of *Mycobacterium tuberculosis* from patients smear-negative for acid-fast bacilli *Lancet* 353(9151):444–449.

Canetti, G. 1962. L' eradication de la tuberculose dans les differents pays, compte-tenudes donditions existantes (problemes theoretiques et solutions pratiques). *Bull Int Union Tuberc Lung Dis* 32:608–642.

Centers for Disease Control and Prevention. 1989. A strategic plan for the elimination of tuberculosis in the United States. *MMWR.* 38:269–272.

Centers for Disease Control and Prevention. 1995. Essential components of a tuberculosis prevention and control program. *MMWR* 44(RR-11):1–16.

Chaulk CP. 1999. Tuberculosis elimination and the challenge of the long-term completer. *Int J Tuberc Lung Dis* 3(4):269.

Communicable Disease Center. 1960. The Arden House Conference on Tuberculosis: November 29, 1959–December 2, 1959. Harriman, NY. Washington, DC: U.S. Department of Health, Education, and Welfare.

Comstock GW, Livesay VT, and Woolpert SF. 1974. The prognosis of a positive tuberculin reaction in childhood and adolescence. *Am J Epidemiol* 99(2):131–138.

Curtis AB, Ridzon R, Vogel R, et al. 1999. Extensive transmission of *Mycobacterium tuberculosis* from a child. *N Engl J Med* 341(20):1539–1540.

Daniel TM, Bates JH, and Downes KA. 1994. History of tuberculosis. In: *Tuberculosis: Pathogenesis, Protection, Control* (Ed. BR Bloom), Washington, DC: ASM Press.

Dubos R, and Dubos J. 1952. *Tuberculosis, Man and Society: The White Plague*. Boston: Little, Brown, and Co.

Etkind SC. 1993. The role of the public health department in tuberculosis control. *Med Clin N Am* 77(6):1303–1314.

Ferebee SH. 1970. Controlled chemoprophylaxis trials in tuberculosis: A general review. *Adv Tuberc Res* 17:28–106.

Frieden TR, Fujiwara PI, Washko RM, and Hamburg MA. 1995. Tuberculosis in New York City—Turning the tide. *N Engl J Med* 333(4):229–233.

Frost W. 1937. How Much Control of Tuberculosis? *Am J Pub Health* 27:759–766.

Grzybowski S, and Allen E. 1964. The challenge of tuberculosis in decline. *Am Rev Respir Dis* 90:5.

Institute of Medicine. 1988. *The Future of Public Health*. Washington, DC: National Academy Press.

International Union Against Tuberculosis Committee on Prophylaxis. 1982. Efficacy of various durations of isoniazid preventive therapy for tuberculosis: Five years of follow-up in the IUAT trial. *Bull WHO* 60(4):555–564.

Mangura BT, Napolitano EC, Passannante MR, McDonald RJ, and Reichman LB. 1998. *Mycobacterium tuberculosis* miniepidemic in a church gospel choir. *Chest* 113(1):234–237.

McGrath JW. 1988. Social networks of disease spread in lower Illinois valley: A simulation approach. *Am J Phys Anthropol* 77:483–496.

Morse D, Brothwell DR, and Ucko PJ. 1964. Tuberculosis in ancient Egypt. *Am Rev Respir Dis* 90:524–541.

Nolan CM, Goldberg S, and Buskin SE. 1999. Hepatotoxicity associated with isoniazid preventive therapy: A 7-year survey from a public health tuberculosis clinic. *JAMA* 281(11):1014–1018.

Palmer C. 1958. Tuberculosis: A decade in retrospect and in prospect. *Lancet* 78:257–260.

Perkins J. 1959. Global eradication of tuberculosis. *Am Rev Respir Dis* 80:138–139.

Reichman LB. 1991. The U-shaped curve of concern. *Am Rev Respir Dis* 144(4):741–742.

Salo WL, Aufderheide AC, Buikstra J, and Holcomb TA. 1994. Identification of *Mycobacterium tuberculosis* DNA in a pre-Columbian Peruvian mummy. *Proc Natl Acad Sci USA* 91:2091–2094.

Shaw JB, and Wynn-Williams N. 1954 Infectivity of pulmonary tuberculosis in relation to sputum status. *Am Rev Tuberc* 69:724–737.

Simone PM, and Fujiwara PI. 1999. Role of the health department—Legal and public health implications. In: *Tuberculosis and Nontuberculous Mycobacterial Infections*, 4th ed. Philadelphia: W.B. Saunders Company, 130–139.

Tabet SR, Goldbaum GM, Hooton TM, Eisenach KD, Cave MD, and Nolan CM. 1994. Restriction fragment length polymorphism analysis detecting a community-based tuberculosis outbreak among persons infected with human immunodeficiency virus. *J Infect Dis* 169(1):189–192.

U.S. Public Health Service. 1944. The Public Health Service Act. *Pub Health Rep* 59:916–919.

Wilson L. 1990. The historical decline of tuberculosis in Europe and America: Its causes and significance. *J History Med Allied Sci* 45:366–396.

2

The Current Situation and How We Got Here

THE HISTORY OF TUBERCULOSIS

Although accurate data that describe the incidence and prevalence of tuberculosis could not have been collected before the identification of *Mycobacterium tuberculosis* by Koch in 1882, "consumption" was well recognized, and deaths thought to be due to the disease were counted for a number of years before its etiology was determined (Koch, 1882). According to Thomas Young, writing in 1815, "The frequency of consumption in Great Britain is usually such that it carries off about one fourth of its inhabitants; at Paris the mortality by consumption has been estimated at one fifth; and at Vienna it is said to be one sixth of the whole. . . ." (Young, 1815). Young also noted that "it [tuberculosis] seems to be most frequent in poor countries, where the inhabitants are ill fed and thinly clothed."

In the United States, tuberculosis accounted for a similar proportion of deaths in large cities during the mid-1800s: 24 percent in Providence, 23 percent in New York, and 15 percent in Philadelphia. As shown in Figure 2-1, mortality rates were of a similar magnitude and followed a similar time course in the United States and Europe, peaking at approximately 400 per 100,000 population in Boston, New York, and Philadelphia combined (Dubos and Dubos, 1952).

The discovery of the etiological agent of tuberculosis provided the fundamental scientific underpinning for programs designed to prevent and control the disease. Organized comprehensive surveillance of mortality from tuberculosis began in the latter part of the 19th century and in the early 20th century although, as indicated in Figure 2-2, data for various

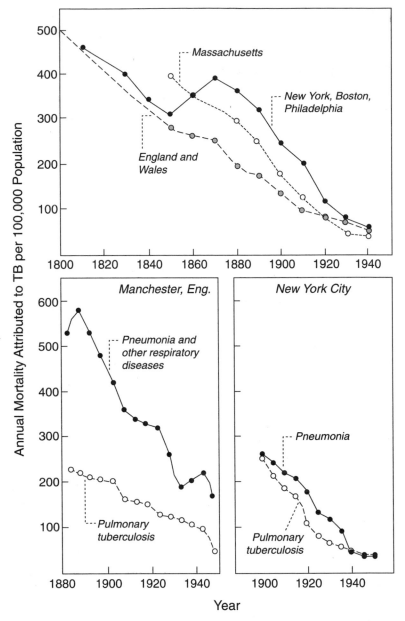

FIGURE 2-1 Dubos, Rene and Jean Dubos, *The White Plague: Tuberculosis, Man, and Society.* Copyright 1952 by Rutgers, The State University. Reprinted by permission of Rutgers University Press.

geographical locales had been collected earlier. These mortality data, although crude, did provide important information about the magnitude of tuberculosis and demonstrated that, generally, rates were declining in advance of the application of any specific control measures. The progressive reduction in mortality rates was sharply and dramatically interrupted by World War I and less dramatically so but also clearly by World War II, as shown in Figure 2-2.

Obviously the equilibrium between man and the tubercle bacillus is very precarious. If war can so rapidly upset it, other unforeseen events might also cause recurrences of the tuberculosis epidemic in the Western World. (Dubos and Dubos, 1952, p. 196)

In the early 1900s the threat of tuberculosis caused by *Mycobacterium bovis* (one of three species in the *Mycobacterium tuberculosis* complex) was also addressed. The Tuberculosis Eradication Division was organized within the U.S. Department of Agriculture Bureau of Animal Industry in 1910 to organize a campaign for the control and eventual elimination of *M. bovis* in cattle to eliminate the threat to humans. This program required that all cattle herds be systematically tuberculin skin tested, that herds with infected cattle be slaughtered (with an indemnity paid to the owner), and that the premises be cleaned and disinfected after the infected animals were removed. This led to a very rapid reduction in the incidence of bovine tuberculosis. Currently, the positive reaction rate among cattle is less than 2 per 1,000 animals, with many of those reactions believed to be false positive. This program has also effectively eliminated tuberculosis in humans because of infection with *M. bovis*. In the late 1970s, an average of only 26 *M. bovis* isolates a year were reported among isolates sent to the Centers for Disease Control (now known as the Centers for Disease Control and Prevention [CDC]); this represents less than 1 percent of the total isolates sent to the CDC each year, and about 0.1 percent of the total number of tuberculosis cases reported each year (Good, 1980). The few new infections that occur seem to be associated with pediatric exposure to infected milk products outside the United States (primarily Mexico) (Danker et al., 1993) and from occupational exposures to infected game and zoo animals (Dalovisio et al., 1992; Fanning and Edwards, 1991; Nation et al., 1999; Thompson et al., 1993). Because of the low risk of disease following infection (Magnus, 1966; Moda et al., 1996), the occupational exposures are also unlikely to result in a barrier to elimination.

Countrywide mortality data for the United States were not available until 1933. Before that time data were collected from state "death registra-

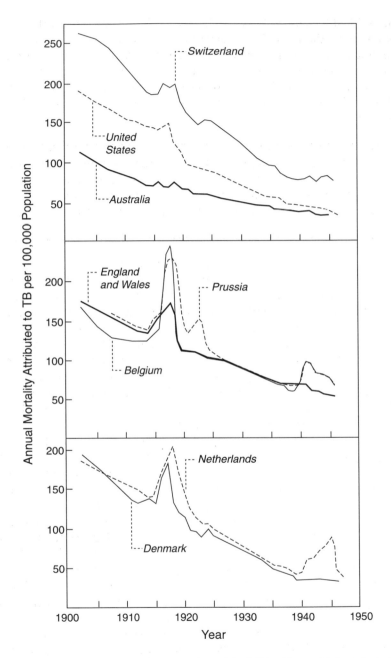

FIGURE 2-2 Dubos, Rene and Jean Dubos, *The White Plague: Tuberculosis, Man, and Society.* Copyright 1952 by Rutgers, The State University. Reprinted by permission of Rutgers University Press.

tion areas," a project that began in 1900 and that comprised eight northeastern states plus Indiana and Michigan. The registration areas gradually expanded so that by 1933 the entire country was included. Tuberculosis morbidity data were also available for the entire continental United States beginning in 1933, when the National Tuberculosis Association (now the American Lung Association) began annual surveys. During the first 20 years of collection of countrywide morbidity data, both active and inactive cases were counted and, as shown in Figure 2-3, the rates declined very little (Centers for Disease Control, 1978). However, beginning in 1953, shortly after the introduction of effective chemotherapy, incidence data began to be collected in much the same way as they are today, with only new active cases being counted. Coincident with the availability of antituberculosis drugs, the rate of decline in tuberculosis mortality rates increased and the incidence of active and inactive cases that had been nearly static for the previous 20 years began to decrease in parallel with the decline in the rate of active cases (Figure 2-3).

From 1953 to 1985 there was, in general, a consistent decline in incidence that averaged 5 to 6 percent per year, resulting in a total reduction of 74 percent, from 84,304 to 22,201 new cases (Figure 2-4). The exceptions to this trend were in 1975, when rates appeared to increase because of a change in reporting criteria, and from 1978 to 1980, when there was an influx of refugees from Southeast Asia, who at that time did not undergo screening or treatment for tuberculosis before they left refugee camps.

CURRENT STATUS OF TUBERCULOSIS

The leveling of the incidence rate curve that began in 1985 followed by the increasing case rates in the late 1980s and early 1990s represented the first true increase in incidence rates since case rate data began to be collected (Figure 2-4). The rate peaked at 10.5 cases per 100,000 population (26,673 cases) in 1992, a 12.9 percent increase over the 1985 rate of 9.3 cases per 100,000 population. The reasons for this increase have not been clearly delineated but are generally thought to be the result of several factors that are both biological and social (Bloom and Murray, 1992). These include the increasing prevalence of human immunodeficiency virus (HIV) infection, increasing rates of homelessness and incarceration, and, perhaps most important, a deterioration in the capacities of tuberculosis control programs to treat patients until cured. Although the natural tendency is for the numbers of tuberculosis cases and deaths from tuberculosis to decline over time, perturbations in various factors, as was seen during the world wars, can cause a reversal in the trend. The observation of René and Jean Dubos (see quote) was prophetic in this regard (Dubos and Dubos, 1952). Although many of the important factors that influence

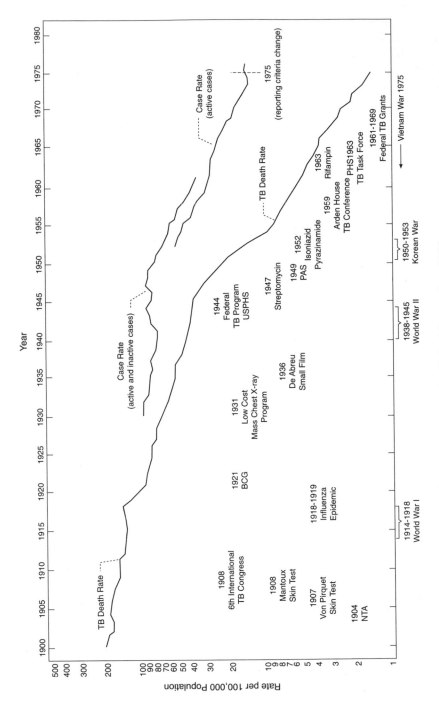

FIGURE 2-3 Tuberculosis case rates and death rates in the United States since 1900.

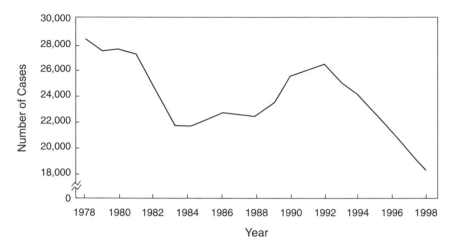

FIGURE 2-4 Reported tuberculosis cases in the United States, 1978–1998.

the incidence of tuberculosis are beyond the control of the public health system, some are well within its control. Because of this tendency for tuberculosis to rebound, given favorable circumstances, the capacity to provide tuberculosis control services must be maintained even in the face of decreasing case rates.

The declines in the numbers of tuberculosis cases and in the case rates that began again in 1993 demonstrate the effectiveness of control measures. However, as will be discussed subsequently, considerably more money was required to regain control of the disease than would have been required previously to maintain control.

The regular decline in tuberculosis case rates that resumed in 1993, reached an all-time low of 6.4 per 100,000 population in 1999 (17,528 cases), for a cumulative 39 percent reduction from the incidence in 1992 (Centers for Disease Control and Prevention, 2000). Just as the reason for the increase in the number of cases was multifactorial, the decrease was as well (Frieden et al., 1995; McKenna et al., 1998). Largely, however, the reduction was caused by a comprehensive strengthening of control activities. A major factor in the resurgence of tuberculosis between 1985 and 1992 was a high frequency of transmission of *M. tuberculosis* within institutions including hospitals, correctional facilities, residential care facilities, and shelters for the homeless population (Daley et al., 1992; Edlin et al., 1992). Since then, improvements in the screening of new entrants to these facilities, more rapid diagnosis, the use of directly observed therapy to decrease infectiousness more rapidly, and more effective use of preventive therapy worked in combination to decrease the number of infectious sources and the potential for transmission. During this period of resurgence, the transmission of M. *tuberculosis* with rapid progression to clinical illness was an important occurrence that was demonstrated by several population-based studies that used molecular epidemiological analyses and that showed unexpectedly high proportions of cases caused by the same strains of the organism (Alland et al., 1994; Small et al., 1994). Conversely, as the number of cases again declined, clustering of cases decreased somewhat disproportionately, suggesting that the measures applied did in fact decrease the level of transmission of the organisms that resulted in rapid progression to disease (Frieden et al., 1995).

During the late 1980s, not only did the number of cases of tuberculosis increase but for the first time large outbreaks caused by M. *tuberculosis* isolates resistant to both isoniazid and rifampin (multidrug-resistant tuberculosis) were recognized (Edlin et al., 1992). A survey of cases from 1982 to 1986 showed that about 0.5 percent of new cases were resistant to both isoniazid and rifampin, but by 1991 the rate of multidrug-resistant tuberculosis had risen to 3.5 percent among all new cases. This increase was the result of a failure to maintain patient adherence with therapy, the use of inappropriate regimens for the treatment of tuberculosis, and system failures, especially slow reporting or the unavailability of laboratory results.

A number of steps were taken to address the problem of multidrug-resistant tuberculosis and these are detailed in the National Action Plan to Combat Multidrug-Resistant Tuberculosis (Centers for Disease Control and Prevention, 1992). Several interventions have been especially important: an emphasis on treating all patients with a four-drug regimen to prevent the emergence of multidrug-resistant tuberculosis in individuals with isoniazid-resistant disease, increased use of directly observed therapy and the application of other patient-centered approaches to promote adherence and completion of therapy, and improved laboratory performance by the use of rapid techniques for the identification of drug-resistant organisms. As a result of these and other measures, the proportion of new cases of multidrug-resistant tuberculosis decreased to 1.1 percent in 1998 (Centers for Disease Control and Prevention, 1999). However, nearly every state in the union has reported at least one case of multidrug-resistant tuberculosis, and it is likely that even if no new cases of multidrug-resistant tuberculosis occur, cases will continue to occur for decades when individuals with latent infection with multidrug-resistant tuberculosis bacilli develop active tuberculosis.

Multidrug-resistant tuberculosis is also a serious problem internationally. The Global Surveillance for Antituberculosis Drug Resistance project, a survey conducted jointly by the International Union Against Tuberculosis and Lung Disease and the World Health Organization found multidrug-resistant tuberculosis in all 52 geographical settings surveyed (World Health Organization, 2000). The estimated proportion of multidrug resistance in previously untreated cases was 1 percent, but the proportions were as high as 10.8 percent in China and 9 percent in Latvia and Russia. The same survey estimated the rate of multidrug resistance among previously treated cases to be 11.1 percent. Given these rates of multidrug-resistant tuberculosis throughout the world and the relatively poor state of global tuberculosis control programs, it is highly likely that there will be continued increases in the proportions and a more widespread distribution of multidrug-resistant cases. Thus, multidrug-resistant tuberculosis presents a threat to the entire world if steps are not taken to cure existing cases and prevent the emergence of new cases.

Recent Incidence Data for the United States

Closer examination of the overall data for the United States in 1998 and 1999 (preliminary data from CDC) reveals a number of important features.

- Tuberculosis increasingly has a heterogeneous distribution. About 75 percent of the new cases occur in the 99 metropolitan areas that have populations of more than 500,000 persons and that account for about 62 percent of the total U.S. population. Nearly half the counties in the United States had no cases of tuberculosis in 1998 (Figure 2-5), although the populations of these counties represented only 11 percent of the total U.S. population. Five states—California, Florida, New York, Illinois, and Texas—had 54 percent of the new cases in 1998, but the decreased incidences in those states also accounted for 68 percent of the overall decrease between 1992 and 1998.
- Tuberculosis is increasingly occurring in foreign-born populations in the United States (Figure 2-6). Although from 1992 to 1999 the number of cases decreased 49 percent among individuals born in the United States, it increased 2 percent among foreign-born persons, and the proportion of individuals with tuberculosis who were born outside of the United States but who now reside in the United States increased from 27 percent in 1992 to 43 percent in 1999. Individuals from three countries—Mexico, the Philippines, and Vietnam—accounted for nearly half of the foreign-born individuals with tuberculosis (23 percent, 13 percent and 10 percent, respectively), with the remaining 54 percent coming from 151 different countries.
- Tuberculosis is relatively common among homeless people or in individuals who reside in congregate facilities, correctional institutions, or long-term-care facilities. Data on the rate of tuberculosis among indi-

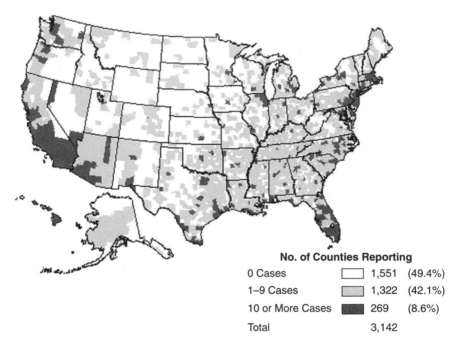

No. of Counties Reporting

0 Cases	☐	1,551	(49.4%)
1–9 Cases	▨	1,322	(42.1%)
10 or More Cases	▰	269	(8.6%)
Total		3,142	

FIGURE 2-5 Reported tuberculosis cases, by county, 1998. SOURCE: CDC.

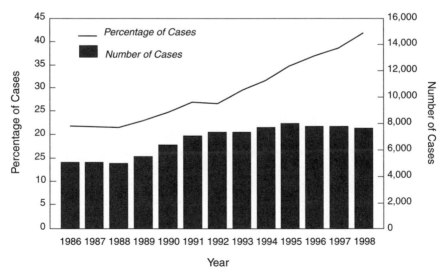

FIGURE 2-6 Trends in tuberculosis cases among foreign-born individuals in the United States (comprising the 50 states, the District of Columbia, and New York City), 1986–1998.

viduals in these populations were not routinely collected before 1993 and were incomplete before the past 2 to 3 years; thus, comparisons of current and previous rates of tuberculosis among individuals in these populations cannot be made. However, nearly 15 percent of the new cases were reported among individuals from what might be considered high-risk environments. Homelessness was an especially prevalent factor among individuals with new cases of tuberculosis in 1997, with, overall, 6.5 percent of the 1997 cases reported as being homeless. In Oregon and the District of Columbia, approximately 17 percent of the new cases, the highest proportions reported, occurred among homeless individuals.

• Substance abuse is common in individuals with tuberculosis. Alcohol abuse was reported in 16.1 percent of the individuals with tuberculosis in 1997, noninjection drug use was reported in 7.8 percent, and injection drug use was reported in 3.3 percent. Again, comparisons with earlier years are not possible.

• The rate of drug resistance, and, particularly, the rate of resistance to isoniazid and rifampin (multidrug resistance), is decreasing. The rate of resistance to isoniazid among new cases decreased from 8.9 percent in 1993 to 8.1 percent in 1998, and the rate of multidrug resistance decreased from 2.8 percent in 1993 to 1.1 percent in 1998. New York and California reported 49 percent of the 150 multidrug-resistant cases. Despite the small number of multidrug-resistant cases, individuals with multidrug-resistant tuberculosis consume a disproportionate amount of the resources in the areas where they live.

• Molecular epidemiological studies have demonstrated that even in efficiently administered tuberculosis control programs, transmission of *M. tuberculosis* from individuals who are acid-fast bacillus smear negative is the cause of at least 15 percent of cases.

Detailed epidemiological analyses such as those described above are essential for determination of the control interventions that have been effective and that are likely to be the most useful in the future. However, similar analyses must also be undertaken at the local level to determine precisely and thoroughly local epidemiological circumstances. In some instances conventional epidemiological analyses can be supplemented by molecular epidemiological analyses to develop an even more precise picture of the local epidemiological circumstances (Hopewell and Small, 1996).

Tuberculosis Control amid Worldwide Complacency

The complacency that was a major factor underlying the resurgence of tuberculosis in the United States, and in many other low-incidence

Tuberculosis and HIV: A Deadly Duo

Throughout both the industrialized and developing world, tuberculosis and HIV disease are closely linked in mutually disadvantageous synergy: HIV infection promotes progression of tuberculosis infection to disease and tuberculosis accelerates the course of HIV disease leading to more opportunistic infections and earlier death. HIV infection greatly increases the likelihood that infection with *Mycobacterium tuberculosis*, either recent or latent, will progress to active tuberculosis. In fact, HIV infection may be the most potent risk factor for tuberculosis yet identified. Conversely, tuberculosis is the most common cause of death in persons with HIV infection throughout the world. The extraordinary, deadly interactions of HIV and *M. tuberculosis* have been amplified by the rapid spread of HIV in populations in which the prevalence of tuberculosis infection was already high. Increasingly, therefore, the control of tuberculosis requires dealing with HIV infection, and vice versa.

Although there are many factors that influence the rate of tuberculosis in persons with HIV infection, data from a multicenter study in the United States showed that, overall, the incidence of tuberculosis was 0.7/100 person years of observation, or slightly less than 1 percent per year. Not surprisingly, rates were higher among those with more severe immune compromise. Among those who had positive tuberculin skin tests the rate was much higher—4.5 per 100 person years. These rates are far in excess of those that would be seen in any comparable group of nonimmunocompromised persons.

While it appears that the impact of HIV infection on the incidence of tuberculosis in the United States is declining, it is quite clear that HIV played a major role in the resurgence of tuberculosis during the late 1980s and early 1990s. At the height of the tuberculosis epidemic in New York City it was estimated that approximately 1/3 of the cases were HIV infected. HIV infection was also a driving force behind the rapid upsurge in cases of tuberculosis caused by multiple drug-resistant organisms (MDR) with much of the transmission occurring in hospitals.

countries as well, was not a new phenomenon. However, the context in which it occurred—a low and progressively declining incidence of disease—was new. In the past the frequency of tuberculosis and, thus, the familiarity that physicians and public health officials have had with the disease have led them to conclude that all that needed to be known about tuberculosis was already known. This was explicitly described by Keers (1978) in his description of the early career of Robert Philip, who in 1887 developed the "Edinburgh Coordinated Scheme," considered to be the first organized effort at the prevention of tuberculosis. According to Keers, "His [Philip's] seniors made it quite clear that they considered tuberculosis to be an exhausted subject. Everything that was to be known about it was already known and understood and every sensible person realized the hopelessness of even thinking about its prevention and treatment" (Keers, 1978).

Although the influence of HIV on the incidence of tuberculosis in the United States is decreasing, data from developing countries indicate a substantial and increasing rate of HIV infection among patients with tuberculosis. In 1992 the World Health Organization (WHO) estimated that worldwide there were approximately 4 million persons who were infected with both *M. tuberculosis* and HIV, nearly 80 percent of these being in Africa. Various studies have reported the prevalence of HIV infection among tuberculosis patients in sub-Saharan African countries to range from 20 to 67 percent. In 1998 the WHO and UNAIDS estimated that of a global total of over 30 million people living with HIV infection, 15 million were coinfected with *M. tuberculosis*, mostly in sub-Saharan Africa. Although this estimate is quite rough, it is indicative of the devastating impact that HIV is having and will continue to have on tuberculosis rates in developing countries.. In Botswana, for example, which has had a model tuberculosis control program using directly observed therapy (DOT) for more than 15 years, the incidence of disease has increased by more than 25 percent since 1995.

On a more positive note, data from many studies demonstrate that tuberculosis in persons with HIV infection responds well to treatment with standard antituberculosis drug regimens. Treatment regimens may, however, be more complicated to manage because of interactions between antiretroviral agents and the drugs used in treating tuberculosis. Even more encouraging is the fact that tuberculosis can be prevented in persons with HIV infection and positive tuberculin skin tests by using any of several proven preventive regimens.

HIV infection is now a fact of life in tuberculosis control. Clearly, any efforts to eliminate tuberculosis must take the effects of HIV infection into account. However, with good tuberculosis control and with effective antiretroviral therapy, the impact of HIV on the incidence of tuberculosis can be greatly reduced. During the past decade a great deal has been learned about both the nature and management of the deadly interaction of *M. tuberculosis* and HIV. This information must now be incorporated into effective interventions for tuberculosis control.

A somewhat paradoxical combination of complacency and defeatism led over the years to a near total dismantling of the World Health Organization's tuberculosis control program. The complacency was manifested as an attitude suggesting that all that was needed for control of tuberculosis was more assiduous application of existing tools at the local level. The defeatism was perhaps best expressed by Walsh and Warren (1979) who, in an analysis of "appropriate" primary health care interventions, concluded that tuberculosis control was too complex and costly to deserve being included as a high-priority activity.

Funding and Mechanisms for Tuberculosis Control in the United States

With the global prevalence of attitudes and the consistently declining rates of tuberculosis in the United States, it is not surprising that funding for domestic tuberculosis programs was progressively eroded to the point that by 1972, no funds from the CDC were specifically directed to tuberculosis control.

Beginning in 1970 the bulk of federal support for tuberculosis control was shifted from a categorical program "(i.e., funds for specific program categories, such as tuberculosis or sexually transmitted diseases), to block grants to the states for control of communicable diseases as a whole, and the states were not required to direct any of the federal funding to tuberculosis (U.S. Congress, Office of Technology Assessment, 1993). The formula by which the amounts of these grants were calculated tended to provide less money to cities of more than 500,000 population (those areas with the highest tuberculosis rates) than had been available under the categorical funding mechanism, also called project grants." Within 2 years of the institution of block grants no categorical money for tuberculosis control was available from the CDC. To compound the problem, there was no way to determine the amounts of the block grants that the states were using for tuberculosis control. The general perception, however, was that funding for tuberculosis control was sharply curtailed.

Categorical funding reappeared via emergency grants in 1980, but as shown in Figure 2-7, this amounted to only $3.6 million in 1980 and $3.7 million in 1981. It was not until 1989 that funding reached the level at which it had peaked in 1969, before the institution of block grants, which

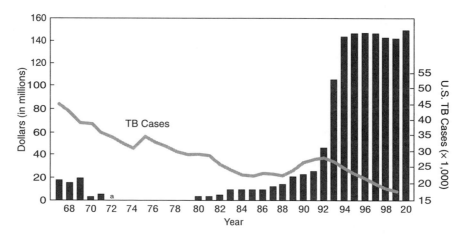

FIGURE 2-7 Tuberculosis funding, Centers for Disease Control and Prevention (CDC), Fiscal Years 1960–1993. NOTE: Categorical grants ceased during Fiscal Years 1972 through 1982; funds to states were in block grants not specific for tuberculosis. SOURCE: Office of Technology Assessment (1993), based on data from the CDC.

was $20 million. The largest increase in federal funding occurred in 1993, the year after case rates peaked, and there was a nearly comparable increase the following year. For the past 6 years (1995 to 2000) funding has been essentially flat at $142 million to $145 million per year. When these amounts are adjusted for inflation, there has been the equivalent of an approximate 15 percent reduction since 1995, the year with peak funding.

Funding at the federal level is only a part of the total financial resources devoted to tuberculosis control. However, because of the highly variable ways in which tuberculosis control activities are supported within states, it is impossible to determine the total amount. In California, for example, funding is from a combination of state and county budgets, as well as from CDC. Other states fund the program entirely from state budgets, usually including CDC support. Large cities are usually responsible for their own programs and received no assistance from the state.

In addition to the support required for public health tuberculosis control programs, other costs arise from the clinical care of patients with tuberculosis. In a comprehensive analysis of the health care expenditures for tuberculosis in the United States, Brown and associates (Brown et al., 1995) estimated that in 1991, direct medical expenditures totaled $703.1 million. Of this, $423.8 million (60 percent) funded inpatient care, a cost not usually borne by tuberculosis control programs. The remaining $279.3 million was expended as follows: $182.3 million for outpatient care, $72.1 million for screening, 3.4 million for contact investigations, $17.9 million for treatment of latent infection, and $3.6 million for surveillance and outbreak investigations. These costs are generally borne by the public health system. In 1991, the year analyzed by Brown and coworkers but not quite the peak year for tuberculosis cases, the amount from CDC for tuberculosis control was $25,274,000, or approximately 10 percent of the estimated countrywide costs, exclusive of inpatient care. If the same relative apportionment of costs is true today, taking into account the fact that in 1998 the number of cases has decreased by 30 percent in 1998 compared to the number in 1991, the costs borne by public health programs for tuberculosis control should have been approximately $195.5 million. If this is true, the $144.5 million provided by CDC represents approximately 74 percent of the public health costs of the disease. Given that the 1991 cost estimates were derived in part from actual data, if relative activity levels have not changed, it would appear that federal funding has largely been used to offset, not to add to, state and local support. However, it is likely that the costs relative to the total number of cases have increased because of the increased use of directly observed therapy, more active screening programs, broader contact investigations, and wider use of treatment of latent infection, all of which are more labor-intensive and, therefore, more costly interventions.

A Dramatic Impact from an Imported Case of Tuberculosis

Young children are rarely suspected of transmitting tuberculosis to adults. Child contacts of individuals with infectious tuberculosis are usually examined to determine if they have been infected by the adult index case patient and to determine if treatment is needed. This conventional wisdom was turned on its head when a woman in North Dakota, who happened to be the guardian of two brothers from the Marshall Islands, was found to have tuberculosis involving her left hip. The two 9-year-old children living with her were examined to determine if they might have been infected by the same source. To the surprise of all involved, one of the brothers was found to have pulmonary tuberculosis with bilateral cavitation on a chest radiograph and sputum specimens strongly positive on smears and by culture. The other brother had a strongly positive tuberculin skin test, a normal chest radiograph, and a single sputum specimen culture that was positive for *M. tuberculosis*. The isolates from the woman and both of the boys all had identical 20-band DNA fingerprints, leading to the conclusion that the 9-year-old child had infected his guardian. Household contact investigations and contact investigation at the primary school attended by the boy resulted in the identification of 120 contacts among 432 individuals screened.

North Dakota is a state with a very low incidence of tuberculosis, with a rate of 1.1 cases per 100,000 population in 1999. In the 5 years before the outbreak described above only one case of tuberculosis in a child under 15 years of age had been reported and only two cases of tuberculosis of any kind had occurred in the two county area in which the woman and the children lived. These cases were, in part, a failure to properly screen the two brothers when they entered the United States. Both received a multiple-puncture tuberculin skin test but the results were not read and they underwent no further screening for tuberculosis. This incident indicates the dramatic impact that a single imported case of tuberculosis can have on a low-incidence community, the importance of screening new arrivals from high-risk areas, and the importance of contact tracing and identification of the source patient. This incident also demonstrates how, as the incidence of tuberculosis declines, conventional wisdom concerning tuberculosis transmission will consistently be challenged and how creative thinking will be needed to identify contacts and manage outbreaks.

SOURCE: Adapted from Curtis et al. (1999).

It is clear that as the number of tuberculosis cases decreases, the costs per case will increase, as long as an adequate infrastructure is maintained. The fixed costs of tuberculosis control are not sensitive to the numbers of cases. Although it is tempting to think that funding can decrease in proportion to the decrease in the number cases, below a certain point (number of cases), reductions cannot be applied without damaging the tuberculosis control infrastructure. In view of the natural history of tuberculosis, generally with a long period of latency between the time of infection and the occurrence of disease, and given that the country has not yet seen the results of the wave of earlier infections, including infections caused by multidrug-resistant organisms that presumably occurred with the resurgence, there is an ongoing, long-term need to maintain effective mechanisms for tuberculosis control. Additional reasons include the fact that it will likely become more difficult to treat patients with tuberculosis because of their social situations and that treatment will require more labor-intensive schemes. Also given the current upheavals in the world, it is likely that the United States will continue to be the destination for large numbers of people from countries with a high incidence of tuberculosis. Even with effective screening, many of these new arrivals will be infected with *M. tuberculosis*. Thus, they may develop tuberculosis at any time in the future.

Maintenance of Control amid Decreased Incidence

A major challenge that needs to be addressed now is how to maintain effective tuberculosis control as the incidence of the disease decreases. This is especially true in parts of the United States where, currently, there are very few cases and a comparably low prevalence of infection. For example, in 1997, seven states had less than 20 new cases each. Yet, outbreaks of tuberculosis may occur in low-incidence areas, such as the outbreak that took place in a rural area along the Kentucky-Tennessee border in 1995 (Valway et al., 1998).

That the downward trend in the number of cases of tuberculosis and the number of deaths from the disease can be reversed by external circumstances has been clearly demonstrated by data from earlier in the 20th century as well as the more recent resurgence. Likewise, the consequences of not having an effective control system in place when unanticipated events occur—for example, the HIV epidemic—recently have been experienced. Although reduced funding was not the only reason for the failure of the system in the late 1980s, it played a major role. It is now necessary to focus on maintenance of an effective control program as the incidence declines and with it the level of concern about tuberculosis.

THE CURRENT LEGAL SYSTEM

Writing in 1993, Lawrence Gostin noted that his survey of state tuberculosis control statutes found "the majority . . . remain antiquated and incompatible with modern standards of constitutional law and public health" (Gostin, 1993, p. 260). Indeed, many statutes were enacted at the turn of the century, and some were enacted in mid-century. Only 10 states had enacted statutes within the previous seven years. Most significantly, the older laws failed to accord individuals with tuberculosis the protections that had increasingly come to characterize the standards applied to those who faced the possible deprivation of liberty. These older statutes had been subjected to judicial review, and characteristic of the deferential posture of the courts to public health enactments for much of the 20th century, they had passed constitutional muster. As late as 1966, a California appellate court had upheld the confinement of a tuberculosis patient pursuant to a law that provided virtually no procedural protections. In its ruling the court declared:

> Health regulations enacted by the state under its police powers and providing even drastic measures for the elimination of disease . . . in a general way are not effected by constitutional provisions either of the state or national government. (Application of Halko, 54 Cal. Report 1966)

This broad deference to the legislature and to the exercise of public health powers would come to look archaic just a few years later as the jurisprudence of confinement underwent a radical revision in the wake of a series of far-reaching constitutional challenges to the power of states to confine patients with psychiatric disorders to mental hospitals. By 1979, Chief Justice Burger would state in *Addington* v. *Texas*:

> The Court has repeatedly recognized that civil commitment for any purpose constitutes a significant deprivation of liberty that requires due process protection. Moreover, it is indisputable that involuntary commitment to a medical hospital . . . can engender adverse social consequences to the individual. Whether we label this phenomena "stigma" or choose to call it something else is less important than that we recognize that it can occur and that it can have a very significant impact on the individual. (*Addington* v. *Texas*, 441 US 418, 425–426 (1979))

Central to constitutional developments was the assertion that before an individual could be deprived of his or her liberty the state had to exhaust other means that were not as intrusive upon the right to liberty. In 1960, the U.S. Supreme Court held in *Shelton* v. *Tucker:*

> Even though the governmental purpose to be legitimate and substantial, that purpose cannot be pursued by means that broadly stifle fundamental personal liberties when the end can be more narrowly achieved. The breadth of legislative abridgment must be viewed in the light of less drastic means for achieving the same basic purpose. (*Shelton* v. *Tucker*, 364 US 479, 488 (1960))

It was on the basis of such developments in mental health law, rather than as a result of challenges to the actions of public health officials in responding to tuberculosis cases, that it became possible to assert successfully that tuberculosis patients be accorded the procedural protections guaranteed by the Constitution. In 1980, in an appellate court decision that upheld the procedural rights of a tuberculosis patient, the Supreme Court of Appeals in West Virginia articulated a standard that expressly followed the developments in mental health law (*Greene* v. *Edwards*, 263 S.E. 2d 661 (W.Va. 1980)). The state's tuberculosis control act was ruled unconstitutional because it did not guarantee the right to counsel, did not provide for the right to cross-examine, confront, and present witnesses, and failed to hold the state to the stringent "clear and convincing" standard of proof required by the U.S. Supreme Court.

The social transformation in the legal and political context within which issues of confinement were considered in the 1970s and 1980s shaped policy and practice in the United States. In 1993, when the Advisory Council for the Elimination of Tuberculosis (ACET) recommended changes in state tuberculosis control laws, it declared

> As in commitment proceedings under state mental health laws, any law under which a person may be examined, isolated, detained, committed and/or treated for TB [tuberculosis] must meet due process and equal protection requirements under state and federal statutes and constitutions. Also, all patients who are subject to these legal proceedings should be represented by legal counsel. (Centers for Disease Control and Prevention, 1993)

Reflecting the doctrine of the least restrictive alternative, the Council recommended, "Before committing TB [tuberculosis] patients for in patient treatment, states should adopt step-by-step interventions beginning with DOT [directly observed therapy] and supplemented by incentives and enablers" (Centers for Disease Control and Prevention, 1993, p. 8).

The Council's incorporation of both procedural due process protections and the doctrine of the least restrictive alternative into its recommendations was especially crucial, because it was calling for the expansion of existing tuberculosis laws to "permit the involuntary isolation and detention of non-infectious patients" who "refuse to adhere to a treatment regimen or to complete treatment" (Centers for Disease Control and Prevention, 1993, p. 8).

This expansion on the conceptions of who posed a threat to the public health, driven by concerns about multidrug-resistant *M. tuberculosis*, represented a move of great significance. No longer did the person to be confined have to represent an immediate threat of transmission. Rather, it was the prospect of reactivation and the prospect of the development of drug resistance that provided the grounds for state intervention. Here the concept of "threat" was informed by the population-based concerns of public health. It was concern about the collective consequence of permitting many individuals to conduct themselves in a way that posed some threat that motivated the extension of public health powers to reach patients who had begun therapy for their tuberculosis but who would not or could not complete their treatment. It was inadequate treatment that posed the threat of multidrug-resistant tuberculosis. This was, however, a calculus far different from one that would center on the potential risk posed by a given individual. Nevertheless, legal commentators have, by and large, agreed that confinement until cure would probably be found constitutional for noninfectious patients who did not adhere to treatment (Bayer and Dupuis, 1995; Gostin, 1995).

A striking reflection of the expansion of the concept of what constitutes a public health threat was the adoption in 1993 of treatment-until-cure regulations by the New York City Board of Health (Ball and Barnes, 1994). The board had concluded "[f]or patients who are unable to complete treatment [until] cure the temporary detention . . . until they are non-infectious is an ineffective public health strategy." Under the newly enacted Section 11.41 of the city's Health Code, the Commissioner of Health could confine an individual for whom there was a "substantial likelihood, based on such person's past and present behavior, that he or she cannot be relied upon" to complete treatment. Under the amended code, a court review had to be accorded to a confined patient within 5 business days, even if the individual did not request release. The Department of Health had to seek judicial review within the first 60 days of detention and subsequently at 90-day intervals. Upon requesting release, the confined individual was entitled to a lawyer and, if too poor to afford counsel, had to be provided with one at public expense. Maryland, too, extended the authority to quarantine tuberculosis patients in the "noncommunicable stage" who "refused to receive sufficient therapy" (Rothenberg and Lovoy, 1994). California extended quarantine authority to non-infectious patients in 1993 and incorporated this into the California Health and Safety Code 121365 in 1994.

Among the controversial elements of the revised New York City code was the way in which the requirements of the least restrictive alternative standard were to be applied. During the hearing process that preceded the adoption of the amended code, civil liberties advocates claimed that the proposed new regulations were unconstitutional because they did not require the city to "exhaust" all less restrictive alternatives before seeking the involuntary confinement of a persistently noncompliant tuberculosis patient.

This broad interpretation of the least restrictive alternative doctrine formed the basis for a constitutional challenge brought against New York City's Health Department in early 1994 (*In re Application of the City of New York v. Doe* No. 40770/94 (1994)). In that challenge, it was argued that a distinction should be made between the latitude that should be available to the Commissioner of Health when confronting a patient with infectious tuberculosis and a noncompliant patient who was not contagious. The distinction between contagious and noncontagious patients was precisely the distinction that the public health authorities concerned about the rise in drug resistance had sought to erase because of the importance of "treatment to cure," regardless of current infectiousness.

Both the extension of procedural protections and the extension of the scope of tuberculosis control to those who are noninfectious have important implications for a policy that is directed at tuberculosis elimination, a centerpiece of which will be identification and treatment of individuals with latent infection. The courts could hold that mandatory screening and treatment represent an unconstitutional extension of the police powers not justified by the level of risk posed by individuals who might decline therapy for latent tuberculosis infection. On the other hand, they could find compelling a public health finding that the elimination of tuberculosis justified the compulsory treatment of latent infection just as the threat of multidrug-resistant tuberculosis justified the imposition of the requirement that those with tuberculosis complete their therapy even though they no longer posed an immediate public health threat.

In commenting on this tension, Lawrence Gostin has noted

> While traditional public health law inquiries focus principally on present infectiousness, there is no reason to limit the direct threat doctrine in this way. . . . Direct threats therefore ought to include significant risks that are reasonably foreseeable. . . . After all, a health department's duty to protect citizens from the risk of foreseeable harm is as strong as its duty to protect citizens from the more imminent risk of infectious transmission. . . . If the state can demonstrate through objective data that the person is likely to develop or reactivate clinically infectious tuberculosis then there is no reason why the state cannot intervene to prevent the future risk to the public. For example, the development of clinically infectious tuberculosis in a person dually infected with HIV and MTB [*M. tuberculosis*] presents a significant risk to fellow residents in a congregate setting. The risk justifies requiring the completion of a course of isoniazid preventive treatment. (Gostin, 1995)

The screening of high-risk populations for latent tuberculosis infection and the provision of treatment of latent infection have been recognized for more than a decade as being central to the goal of tuberculosis elimination. First priority in such efforts must be given to those at highest risk—those recently exposed to tuberculosis, contacts of individuals with suspected or confirmed cases of tuberculosis, and patients with or at risk for HIV infection.

THE REALITY OF ELIMINATION

"Elimination," as applied to infectious diseases, has been defined in many different ways, including reduction of the incidence, prevalence, morbidity, mortality, or transmission of a disease or of the pathogen that causes it. Often, especially since the successful eradication of smallpox, the word "elimination" has been used deliberately to invoke the cachet of *eradication* in circumstances in which the goal of true eradication is known to be unattainable. Such use of the term "elimination" is thus designed to mislead by implying one thing, that is, eradication, while really denoting something else, namely, a goal that is different from eradication. Even the potential distinctions between "elimination" and "eradication" in English are lost in some other languages that use only one word that means eradication and that is equivalent in meaning to both English words. Inappropriate, indiscriminate, or promiscuous use of "elimination" and "eradication" causes confusion and risks devaluing the legitimate concept of disease eradication among the general public and lay policy makers.

In 1997, a group of scientists who met in Dahlem (Berlin), Germany, for a week to consider aspects of the eradication of infectious diseases proposed that *elimination of disease* be defined as "reduction to zero of the incidence of a specified disease in a defined geographic area as a result of deliberate efforts; continued intervention measures are required" (because the same disease might still exist somewhere else). *Elimination of infection* was defined as "reduction to zero of the incidence of infection caused by a specific agent in a defined geographic area as a result of deliberate efforts; continued measures to prevent the reestablishment of transmission are required." *Eradication* was defined to indicate "permanent reduction to zero of the worldwide incidence of infection caused by a specific agent as a result of deliberate efforts," whereas *control* referred to "reduction of disease incidence, prevalence, morbidity or mortality to a locally acceptable level as a result of deliberate efforts" (Dowdle and Hopkins, 1998). The scientists at Dahlem did not evaluate various infectious diseases as to their eradicability or whether they could reasonably be targeted for eradication, elimination or control.

In 1989, the CDC and the ACET published a strategic plan that articulated a national goal to reduce the incidence of tuberculosis to 3.5 cases per 100,000 population by the year 2000 and to less than 1 case per 1 million population by 2010. This goal was called "elimination of tuberculosis" (in the United States). Although the stated goal qualifies use of "elimination" by specifying a quantified target level of disease incidence, that stated goal does not meet the criteria for elimination suggested by the Dahlem Conference. By the Dahlem Conference criteria, the CDC-ACET target is a goal of tuberculosis *control*.

Ironically, the CDC-ACET goal was promulgated during a period when case rates were not declining, and in the following year an unexpected upsurge in the incidence of tuberculosis ensued in the United States. Instead of the steady decline in the number of cases by about 7 percent per year that had occurred before 1985, the number of new cases of tuberculosis in the United States increased from 22,201 in 1985 to 26,673 in 1992. Since 1992, however, tuberculosis incidence in the United States has resumed its decline, again at a rate of about 6 percent per year, to 17,528 new cases in 1999, or 6.4 cases per 100,000 population. Thus, the 1999 U.S. incidence (6.4 per 100,000 population) is almost twice the stated goal for 2000 (3.5 per 100,000 population). At the current rate of decline, the U.S.'s case rate of tuberculosis would reach the stated goal for 2010 (1 per 1 million population) only after about 60 more years. If the current rate of reduction in annual incidence were doubled, which is imaginable by use of current tuberculosis control tools, it would still take about 27 years to reach the target of "elimination." Achievement of the current target of 1 case per 1 million population in the United States by the target year of 2010 would require an average annual rate of decline of 32 percent.

The current Institute of Medicine committee endorses the general concept of "elimination" of tuberculosis in the United States as rapidly as feasible. However, the committee stresses the urgent need to accelerate the annual rate of reduction in the incidence of the disease by better use of the tools that are already available and by development of more effective tools to reduce the risk of transmission of the infection and to reduce the risk of development of the disease by those already infected in the United States. Accelerating the annual rate of decline of tuberculosis in the United States also requires that more attention be given to assisting with tuberculosis control efforts in a few countries that are the sources of the most cases imported into the United States. Any relaxation of current efforts against tuberculosis in the United States risks another resurgence in the disease and the potential loss of hard-won gains. Acceleration of the rate of reduction in the incidence of new cases is important for the following reasons:

- It would reduce the suffering of individuals with tuberculosis.
- It would reduce the costs of medical care for such patients.
- It would reduce the risk of resurgence of the disease.
- It would reduce the risk of multidrug-resistant cases.
- It would reduce the risk of spread of cases to tuberculosis-free areas of the United States.
- It would reduce the complications caused by tuberculosis in HIV-infected individuals.

• It would lead and contribute to reduction in the global burden of tuberculosis.

• It would hasten the eventual elimination of tuberculosis from the United States.

Successful eradication programs have used a few key indicators to monitor progress toward their ultimate objective. The committee recommends the use of a few such key indicators to monitor and to regularly report on progress related to defined, quantitative targets and interim benchmarks for the tuberculosis elimination program. The development of these indicators will require a better understanding of the epidemiology as it approaches elimination.

THE ETHICS OF TUBERCULOSIS ELIMINATION

With the incidence and prevalence of tuberculosis declining to the lowest levels in history in the United States and with the burden of tuberculosis continuing to exact an enormous toll in less developed nations, the ethical challenges posed by the goal of tuberculosis elimination are neither simple nor straightforward. In the United States, federal, state, and local governments have the moral duty to fund tuberculosis control programs so that every case of tuberculosis is promptly identified and every patient is treated until he or she is cured. The experience of the past decade has demonstrated the price to be paid in morbidity and mortality when such efforts are less than adequate. There is no justification for repeating the cycle of concern and neglect. The past decade has also demonstrated the necessity of using a range of strategies to ensure that treatment completion rates of 90 percent and better are sustained. Both ethical principles and constitutional standards require that the least restrictive measures that can be effective be used to achieve that end. Social supports and incentives for those patients are essential. Recourse to liberty-depriving measures may be necessary but should be viewed as a last resort and should be relied upon only after a hearing before a tribunal where the rights of the individual are given due accord.

The goal of tuberculosis elimination, however, will require more than case finding and treatment. It is now clear that an increasing focus on the identification and treatment of individuals with latent infections will be essential. It is in this regard that the ethical challenges will be new and difficult. How should individuals with latent tuberculosis infection be identified? From an epidemiological perspective, it is clear that targeted screening efforts are more efficient than those that cast a net that includes individuals at very low risk. However, can targeting efforts be undertaken without the taint of stigmatization? This is a question that is bound to arise since those at greatest risk are also poor, vulnerable, and marginalized.

More difficult still is the question of whether such screening should be voluntary, undertaken with the cooperation of various community-backed organizations that can effectively encourage those at risk to be tested for latent infection, or should be compulsory.

There is little question that in selected settings screening for active tuberculosis can be undertaken on a compulsory basis. The constitutional authority granted under the police powers of the state has been used to justify such efforts. From an ethical perspective, the concept of the harm principle justifies state intervention when an individual places others at risk. Are these doctrines and principles, however, sufficiently robust to justify mandatory screening for latent infection that poses only the *prospect* of a public health threat? Are the constitutional doctrines that, since early in the 20th century, have recognized the authority of the state to impose vaccination requirements to prevent disease sufficiently robust to justify mandatory screening for those at risk for disease?

Finally, there is the question of whether those who are identified to have latent infection should be encouraged to undergo treatment or should be required to do so. The answer to this question very much depends on the risks involved in both the decision to treat and the decision not to treat and the benefits to both the individual and the public health from the initiation and completion of treatment of latent infection. The consistency with which treatment of latent infection is now recommended makes it clear that, with the exception of those in whom treatment is clinically contraindicated, the weight of medical authority now supports treatment. Even when treatment is clearly beneficial, however, the traditions of informed consent derived from constitutional doctrines and the ethical principle of autonomy typically dictate that competent adults be free to choose whether or not to undergo therapy. Even in the context of those committed to a hospital on psychiatric grounds, the courts have held that the decision to impose therapy against the wishes of the patient requires a special hearing.

On the other hand, the courts have long recognized the right of the state to require treatment for infectious diseases such as tuberculosis that pose a public health threat. Furthermore, in the early 1990s, a number of jurisdictions recognized that the authority to treat infectious tuberculosis was sufficiently robust to justify the requirement that patients in whom tuberculosis was no longer infectious undergo treatment until cure. Does the extension of the scope of the state's public health authority to individuals who pose only a potential threat provide the justification for mandatory therapy for individuals with latent infection? Do different contexts defined in terms of a heightened risk of transmission, were actual disease to develop, help to identify those settings within which mandatory treatment for latent infection would be justifiable? Do, for example, the unique features of homeless shelters or prisons justify mandatory treatment that would otherwise raise constitutional and ethical questions? As discussed further in Chapter 4, the conclusion of this committee is that the answer to all of these questions is yes. However, the committee was also cognizant of the social vulnerability of these populations and the need to protect against unnecessary coercion of the powerless.

The issues of screening and treatment for latent infection compel society to address the questions of when, if ever, it is appropriate to use compulsory public health powers and how to balance the collective well-being against the right of the individual to be free of intrusions when the threat that he or she poses to others is only statistical. These issues take on special significance in the context of the goal of tuberculosis elimination.

The ethical challenges posed by the continued burden of tuberculosis in less developed nations are very different. It is possible to argue that, on the grounds of narrow self-interest, the United States and other developed nations should be concerned with tuberculosis abroad because it is not possible to erect a protective cordon sanitaire. This is especially the case with tuberculosis at the border, as is the case with Mexico and the United States. To so frame the issue, however, is to unduly restrict the U.S. moral vision. Eight million cases of tuberculosis annually worldwide and 2 million to 3 million deaths a year demand attention, regardless of their ultimate impact on American well-being. The United States shares with other developed nations the obligation to shoulder the task of fostering the development of a tuberculosis vaccine as well as new diagnostic tests and drugs. Only the developed nations have the scientific, technological, and financial resources necessary to make possible the long-term effort that vaccine development will especially require. It is that capacity that imposes the moral duty on developed nations to act to save the lives of millions who would otherwise die.

The ethical duty to rescue those who might otherwise fall victim to tuberculosis requires that the developed nations provide the resource commitment that can effectively be used. Ongoing scientific analysis of the extent to which resource constraints are hindering efforts at vaccine development are critical. Although there is no justification for expending resources that cannot be reasonably used, neither is there a justification for spending less than can productively be invested.

REFERENCES

Addington v. Texas 441 U.S. 418, 425–426 (1979).

Alland D, Kalkut GE, Moss AR, et al. 1994. Transmission of tuberculosis in New York City: An analysis by DNA fingerprinting and conventional epidemiologic methods. N Engl J Med 330(24):1710–1716.

Ball CA, and Barnes M. 1994. Public health and individual rights: Tuberculosis control and detention procedures in New York City. Yale Law Pol Rev 12:38–67.

Bayer, R., Dupuis, L., 1995. Tuberculosis, Public Health, and Civil Liberties. Annual Review of Public Health 16: 307–26.

Bloom BR, and Murray CJ. 1992. Tuberculosis: Commentary on a reemergent killer. Science 257(5073):1055–1064.

Brown RE, Miller B, Taylor WR, et al. 1995. Health-care expenditures for tuberculosis in the United States. Arch Intern Med 155(15):1595–1600.

Centers for Disease Control and Prevention. 1978. Extrapulmonary Tuberculosis in the United States (Pub. No. USPHS/CDC 78-8360). Atlanta: CDC.

Centers for Disease Control and Prevention. 1992. National action plan to combat multidrug-resistant tuberculosis. MMWR 41(RR-11):5–48.

Centers for Disease Control and Prevention. 1993. Tuberculosis control laws—United States, 1993. Recommendations of the Advisory Council for the Elimination of Tuberculosis. MMWR 42(Suppl. RR-15):1–28.

Centers for Disease Control and Prevention 2000. Reported Tuberculosis in the United States, 1998. Atlanta: CDC.

Curtis, AB, Ridzon R, Vogel R, et al. 1999. Extensive transmission of Mycobacterium tuberculosis from a child. N Engl J Med 341:1491–1495.

Daley CL, Small PM, Schecter GF, et al. 1992. An outbreak of tuberculosis with accelerated progression among persons infected with the human immunodeficiency virus: An analysis using restriction-fragment-length polymorphisms. N Engl J Med 326(4):231–235.

Dalovisio JR, Stetter M, and Mikota-Wells S. 1992 Rhinoceros Rhinorrhea: Cause of an outbreak of infection due to airborne Mycobacterium bovis in zookeepers. Clin Infect Dis 15:598–600.

Danker WM, Waecker NJ, Essey MA, Moser K, Thompson M, and Davis CE. 1993. Mycobacterium bovis infections in San Diego: A clinicoepidemiologic study of 73 patients and a historical review of a forgotten pathogen. Medicine 77:11–37.

Dowdle WR, and Hopkins DR (eds.). 1998. The Eradication of Infectious Diseases. New York: John Wiley & Sons.

Dubos R, and Dubos J. 1952. Tuberculosis, Man and Society: The White Plague. New Brunswick, NJ: Rutgers University Press.

Edlin BR, Tokars JI, Grieco MH, et al. 1992. An outbreak of multidrug-resistant tuberculosis among hospitalized patients with the acquired immunodeficiency syndrome. N Engl J Med 326(23):1514–1521.

Fanning A, and Edwards S. 1991. Mycobacterium bovis infection in human beings in contact with elk (Cervus elaphus) in Alberta, Canada. The Lancet 338:1253–1255.

Frieden TR, Fujiwara PI, Washko RM, and Hamburg MA. 1995. Tuberculosis in New York City—Turning the tide. N Engl J Med 333(4):229–233.

Good RC. 1980. Isolation of nontuberculous mycobacteria in the United States, 1979. J Infect Dis 142(5):779–783.

Gostin, L. 1993. Controlling the resurgent tuberculosis epidemic: A 50-state survey of TB statutes and proposals from reform. J Am Med Assoc 269:255–261.

Gostin L. 1995. The resurgent tuberculosis epidemic in the era of AIDS: Reflections on public health, law and society. Maryland Law Rev 54:1–131.

Greene v. *Edwards* 263 S.E. 2d 661 (W. Va. 1980).

Hopewell PC, and Small PM. 1996. Applications of Molecular Epidemiology to the Prevention, Control, and Study of Tuberculosis. In: *Tuberculosis* (Eds. Rom WM, and Garay S). Boston: Little, Brown, and Co., pp. 113–127.

In re *Application of the City of New York* v. *Doe* (No. 40770/94) (1994).

Keers RY. 1978. *Pulmonary Tuberculosis: A Journey Down the Centuries*. London: Balliere-Tindall.

Koch R. 1882. Die Ätiologie der Tuberkulose. *Berliner Klinischen Wchenschrift* 15:221–230.

Magnus K. 1966. Epidemiological basis of tuberculosis eradication. 3. Risk of pulmonary tuberculosis after human and bovine infection. *Bull World Health Org* 35:483–508.

McKenna MT, McCray E, Jones JL, Onorato IM, and Castro KG. 1998. The fall after the rise: Tuberculosis in the United States, 1991 through 1994. *Am J Pub Health* 88(7):1059–1063.

Moda G, Daborn CJ, Grange JM, and Cosivi O. 1996. The zoonotic importance of *Mycobacterium bovis*. *Tubercl Lung Dis* 77:103–108.

Nation PN, Fanning EA, Hopf HB, and Church TL. 1999. Observations on animal and human health during the outbreak of *Mycobacterium bovis* in game farm Wapiti in Alberta. *Can Vet J* 40:113–117.

Rothenberg KH, and Lovoy EC. 1994. Something old, something new: The challenge of tuberculosis control in the age of AIDS. *Buffalo Law Rev* 42:715–760.

Small PM, Hopewell PC, Singh SP, et al. 1994. The epidemiology of tuberculosis in San Francisco: A population-based study using conventional and molecular methods. *N Engl J Med* 330(24):1703–1709.

Shelton v. *Tucker* 364 U.S. 479, 488 (1960).

Thompson et al. 1993. Seals, seal trainers, and mycobacterial infectionl. *Am Rev Respir Dis* 147:164–167.

U.S. Congress, Office of Technology Assessment (OTA). 1993. The continuing challenge of tuberculosis. (Pub. No. OTA-H-574). Washington, DC: OTA.

Valway SE, Sanchez MPC, Shinnick TF, et al. 1998. An outbreak involving extensive transmission of a virulent strain of *Mycobacteium tuberculosis*. *N Engl J Med* 338(10):633–639.

Walsh JA, and Warren KS. 1979. Selective primary health care: An interim strategy for disease control in developing countries. *N Engl J Med* 301(18):967–974.

World Health Organization/International Union Against Tuberculosis. *2000 Global Project on Anti-Tuberculosis Drug Resistance Surveillance* (Rep. No. 2). Geneva, Switzerland: Author.

Young T. 1815. *A Practical and Historical Treatise on Consumptive Disease*. London.

3

Tuberculosis Elimination and the Changing Role of Tuberculosis Control Programs

The steady decline in the incidence of tuberculosis over the last 8 years indicates that the disease is once again under control in the United States, but a number of challenges lie ahead if control is to be maintained. Declining numbers of cases will pose challenges in maintaining the expertise necessary for tuberculosis control and could result in premature decreases in tuberculosis control budgets. At the same time health care delivery systems are changing, as there is a trend toward increased privatization of health care and social services and increased use of managed care organizations for the delivery of services. All of these challenges can also create opportunities. This chapter reviews the changes that lie ahead and outlines strategies for maintaining the decline in the incidence of tuberculosis.

RECOMMENDATIONS

Recommendation 3.1 To permanently interrupt the transmission of tuberculosis and prevent the emergence of multidrug-resistant tuberculosis, the committee recommends that

• **All states have health regulations that mandate completion of therapy (treatment to cure) for all patients with active tuberculosis.**
• **All treatment be administered in the context of patient-centered programs that are based on individual patient characteristics. Such programs must be the standard of care for patients with tuberculosis in all settings.**

Recommendation 3.2 To ensure the most efficient application of existing resources, the committee recommends that

• New program standards be developed and used by the Centers for Disease Control and Prevention (CDC) and state and local health departments to evaluate program performance.

• Standardized, flexible case management systems be developed to provide the information needed for the evaluation measurements. These systems should be integrated with existing case management systems and other automated public health data systems whenever possible.

Recommendation 3.3 To make further progress toward the elimination of tuberculosis in regions of the country experiencing low rates of disease, the committee recommends that

• Tuberculosis elimination activities be regionalized through a combination of federal and multistate initiatives to provide better access to and more efficient utilization of clinical, epidemiological, and other technical services.

• Protocols and action plans be developed jointly by CDC and the states for use by state and local health departments to enable planning for the availability of adequate resources.

• State and local health departments develop case management plans to ensure a uniform high quality of care for patients with tuberculosis and tuberculosis infection in their jurisdictions.

Recommendation 3.4 To maintain quality in tuberculosis care and control services in an era of increased use of managed care systems and privatization of services, the committee recommends that

• When it is determined that tuberculosis treatment can be provided more efficiently outside of the public health department, the delivery of such services be governed by well-designed contracts that specify performance measures and responsibilities.

• Federal categorical funding for tuberculosis control be retained. Funding at the local level should provide sufficient dedicated resources for tuberculosis control but should be structured to provide maximum flexibility and efficiency.

• Both public and private health insurance programs be billed for tuberculosis diagnostic and treatment services whenever possible but tuberculosis services should never be denied due to a patient's inability to make a co-payment.

Recommendation 3.5 To promote a well-trained medical (in a broad sense) workforce and educated public, the committee recommends that

   • **The Strategic Plan for Tuberculosis Training and Education, which contains the blueprint that addresses the training and educational needs for tuberculosis control, be fully funded.**
   • **Programs for the education of patients with tuberculosis be developed and funded.**
   • **Funding be provided for government, academic, and nongovernmental agencies to work in collaboration with international partners to develop training and educational materials.**

BACKGROUND

The future of tuberculosis in the United States is dependent on not one but two competing races to elimination. The first is the race to reduce the incidence of tuberculosis by implementing measures to stop both transmission and reactivation of the disease. As the number of tuberculosis cases declines, however, only the very optimistic could believe that resources for tuberculosis control will, as a matter of course, be protected. Instead, a second race seems likely—one of elimination of local, state, and federal public health tuberculosis control resources by reallocation of those resources to competing priorities. Tuberculosis elimination is dependent on the results of this second race, with the best outcome being that it is never run. Strategies to that end include not only aggressive promotion of the vision of tuberculosis elimination but also continual adaptation and evolution of the tuberculosis control program response to an increasingly uncommon disease.

What factors should be considered to make this evolution of programs as productive as possible?

The key goals of a successful tuberculosis control program are not controversial. They have been well articulated by the Advisory Council for the Elimination of Tuberculosis and consist of the following:

1. Identify and treat individuals with active tuberculosis.

2. Find and test individuals who have had contact with tuberculosis patients to determine whether they are infected. If they are, provide appropriate treatment.

3. Screen populations at risk for infection to detect infected individuals and provide therapy to prevent progression.

Progress toward tuberculosis elimination will not change these goals. Although the federal government provides substantial resources and technical assistance for public health activities, under the Constitution, states, as the repository of powers not specifically delegated to the federal government, have the responsibility for the health of their citizens. For public health, these responsibilities have been well defined in the Institute of Medicine (1988) report *The Future of Public Health.* As applied to tuberculosis control programs these responsibilities include

- *assessment,* through regular and systematic collection and analysis of information about the extent of tuberculosis infection and disease in a community and the effectiveness of programs and interventions that will reduce this threat;
- *policy development,* through comprehensive, evidence-based policy formulation that allows equitable and effective distribution of public tuberculosis control resources and complementary private activities; and
- *assurance* that services necessary to achieve tuberculosis control are provided by encouraging and enabling actions by other entities, by requiring such actions through regulation, or by providing services directly.

As with tuberculosis control goals, these core functions of tuberculosis control programs will not change as the country moves toward tuberculosis elimination.

CHANGES IN TUBERCULOSIS CONTROL PROGRAM STRATEGIES

Although tuberculosis control goals and core public health functions are fixed, the strategies that emerge from linking the two are not. Instead, these strategies will be influenced by the two effects of moving toward tuberculosis elimination: declining numbers of cases and competition for tuberculosis control resources. This section discusses the nature of these effects and suggests steps that tuberculosis control programs can take to anticipate and plan for them. Not all tuberculosis control programs will adapt to declining numbers of cases at the same pace. Each program should be guided by the local situation, including the extent to which tuberculosis elimination is becoming a local reality. Key elements of effective tuberculosis control programs (for example, sophisticated public tuberculosis clinics or categorical outreach workers) in relatively high-incidence areas will be justified long after they have been abandoned in other low-incidence areas. Jurisdictions experiencing declining rates of tuberculosis, however, must periodically reassess their approaches to the three tuberculosis control goals.

Identify and Treat Individuals with Active Tuberculosis

Traceable partially to sound reasoning of the sanatorium era and partially to tradition, the public health approach to the medical treatment of tuberculosis is unique. Without question, improperly treated tuberculosis poses a risk to society, and as a consequence, tuberculosis control programs must ensure that persons with tuberculosis receive appropriate therapy. For no other disease, however, has this assurance function been translated into so much primary responsibility for the direct provision of medical treatment by the public health system. Data from CDC annual reports on tuberculosis show that since 1993 slightly less than one-half of all tuberculosis patients are treated by health departments and about one-quarter each are either managed by private providers or comanaged by private-sector providers and the health department. It is common for those patients being comanaged to receive medication from the health department; thus, nearly three-quarters of all patients receive medications from their health departments.

A primary argument for direct provision of care in health department tuberculosis clinics has been that treatment of tuberculosis is complex and specialized and requires experience (Sbarbaro, 1970). In high-incidence areas, well-functioning public tuberculosis clinics with competent staff serving most patients with tuberculosis are a valuable element of national tuberculosis control. In many jurisdictions, however, as tuberculosis case counts decline, the "experience" rationale for a public health tuberculosis clinic will become increasingly inapplicable and at some point will be outweighed by the costs of this approach. These costs include the increasing inefficiency of maintaining a clinic and a staff capable of providing tuberculosis services as patient loads drop and become increasingly unpredictable. As importantly, perhaps, these costs also include the opportunity costs incurred by focusing scarce tuberculosis control resources on the direct provision of services. The *Future of Public Health* report observes:

> The direct provision by health departments of personal health services to patients who are unwanted by the private sector absorbs so much of the limited resources available to public health—money, human resources, energy, time, and attention—that the price is higher than it appears. (Institute of Medicine, 1988, p. 52)

As outlined in Chapter 4, tuberculosis elimination will require increased attention to communitywide screening and to the treatment of those with latent infections. Unwarranted attention to the direct provision of medical services for the treatment of active disease must not stop the prevention of cases through the treatment of latent infection from become an increasing focus of state and local tuberculosis control programs.

Instead, as the numbers of cases decline, jurisdictions that directly provide diagnostic and treatment services to individuals with active disease should continually assess the costs and benefits of this approach. In many areas, declining numbers of cases and shifting priorities will likely result in an increasing reliance on the alternative: ensuring that most or all of these services are provided in the private sector. This shift is already beginning. In Missouri, for example, the state tuberculosis control program has identified and contracted with 80 private providers in rural areas to provide services to uninsured patients with tuberculosis. The Tacoma/Pierce County Health Department has contracted with a private group of infectious disease specialists to provide diagnostic and treatment services for all patients with active tuberculosis. This model is described in the box, A Cooperative Public-Private Model for Tuberculosis Control.

Assurance of provision of services in the private sector is not a perfect solution. Public-sector tuberculosis control programs still have the responsibility to ensure that patients are receiving appropriate treatment by monitoring patients on a case-by-case basis. The resources and competence required to provide this assurance function must be available. The extent to which the private sector is up to the task, particularly with respect to the provision of directly observed therapy, is still a subject of debate. However, unpublished data from CDC show that from 1993 to 1997 the proportion of patients who completed therapy within one year when a year or less of therapy was indicated steadily increased both for patients managed by private providers and for patients managed by the health departments. In 1997, 81 percent of patients managed by health departments completed therapy, whereas 77 percent of the patients managed by private providers completed therapy, a possibly important but not large difference.

Objectively, the case can be made that tuberculosis diagnostic and therapeutic considerations are not all that difficult relative to those of other complex medical conditions routinely managed by the private sector. In fact, it is possible that the traditional public health approach of assuming direct responsibility for tuberculosis treatment has enabled the disconnection between the private sector and tuberculosis treatment. The increasing shift to managed care in the United States along with the potential ability and interest of managed care to provide the services required for appropriate care for tuberculosis may facilitate this transition. In the final analysis, the debate over whether the private sector is ready may be moot. In many areas, economies of scale are forcing the abolishment of standalone public-sector tuberculosis clinics and may dictate the integration of this activity into a comprehensive medical practice able to provide this as one of many services.

There is a major conceptual and philosophical difference, however, between the public and private sectors when it comes to treatment, and that difference relates to the locus of responsibility for the successful completion of therapy. The responsibility for successful treatment of the patient with tuberculosis rests with the provider rather than the patient. Although the patient cannot be absolved of responsibility, ultimately treatment failure is provider failure. Although treatment of, for example, diabetes or hypertension is both more complex than treatment of tuberculosis and lifelong, the benefits of such treatment largely accrue to the patient. With treatment of tuberculosis the benefits of successful therapy accrue both to the patient and to society. Moreover, treatment failure often leads to drug resistance, thus decreasing the chances for cure and greatly increasing the costs. Therefore, successful treatment of tuberculosis is a societal imperative as well as a benefit to an individual's health. Once the responsibility for successful treatment has been realized and accepted by the provider, exactly how the goal is achieved is somewhat secondary.

Find and Test Individuals Who Have Had Contact with Tuberculosis Patients to Determine Whether They Are Infected: If They Are, Provide Appropriate Treatment

The declining incidence of tuberculosis will also result in less local experience in conducting case investigations and contact identification and follow-up. In contrast to the provision of diagnostic treatment services to patients with tuberculosis, however, tuberculosis control programs will continue to have direct responsibility for conducting case investigation and contact identification and follow-up, as there is no other appropriate provider of services. The key challenge posed by progress to tuberculosis elimination will be to maintain competency and to develop strategies for ensuring that resources for tuberculosis elimination are available, despite a diminishing and unpredictable demand for services. The complexity and sophistication of these investigations will increase. This area is directly addressed later in the report.

Screen Populations at Risk for Infection to Detect Infected Individuals and Provide Therapy to Prevent Progression

A primary thesis of this report is that successful elimination of tuberculosis will require much greater attention to the screening of at-risk populations. The notion that the reservoir of people with latent infection

A Cooperative Public-Private Model for Tuberculosis Control

Pierce County, in the state of Washington, has a population of 735,000, and Tacoma, with a population of about 195,000, is its largest city. In 1999 the county reported 43 cases of tuberculosis for a rate 5.9 per 100,000 population, compared with the national rate of 6.8 per 100,000. The population of the county has changed from 16 percent nonwhite in 1990 to 24 percent nonwhite in 2000, and the largest component of this population change consists of immigrant from Southeast Asia and the Pacific Islands. Reflecting this change, the proportion of foreign-born individuals with tuberculosis in Pierce County has been about 50 percent over the past year, which is somewhat higher than the proportion of 41 percent foreign-born individuals with tuberculosis for the United States as a whole. There has been one case of multidrug-resistant tuberculosis in the last 5 years, and most years the proportion of isoniazid-resistant cases runs about 12 percent. In general the epidemiological picture of tuberculosis in Pierce County is very similar to that in most parts of the United States with moderate to low rates of tuberculosis.

Until 1996 the provision of medical care for tuberculosis and tuberculosis control services in Pierce County were typical of that in most of the rest of the United States. The County Health Department operated a tuberculosis clinic that received referrals from private providers in the county. The clinic was staffed by a part-time pulmonary specialist who evaluated all patients with tuberculosis and a public health nursing staff that provided clinical follow-up, contact tracing, and tuberculin skin testing and that maintained statistics on the rates and characteristics of tuberculosis in the county. An outreach staff provided directly observed therapy. The public health nurse was also responsible for contact tracing, screening high-risk individuals for tuberculosis infection, and maintaining tuberculosis control statistics for the county.

In 1996, motivated in large part by the Institute of Medicine report on *The Future of Public Health* (Institute of Medicine, 1988) and a desire to improve services while decreasing costs, the health department director and the Board of Health decided to contract out clinical care services for patients with tuberculosis. Following a competitive bidding process, a contract between the Board of

must be actively treated instead of the notion that society should passively wait for infected individuals to die or develop disease must be embraced by tuberculosis control staff and, in turn, promoted to public health policy makers and the practicing medical community in a convincing manner. For most areas, this activity will involve both qualitative and quantitative increases in efforts over current efforts and will require new or redirected resources. The American Thoracic Society (ATS) and CDC have published new guidelines for these efforts (American Thoracic Society, 2000). These guidelines call for targeted tuberculin skin testing of populations at high risk of infection and the treatment of latent infections for all those found to be infected. The guidelines also introduce short-

Health and Infections Limited, a group of infectious disease specialists, was signed in October 1996. The contract provides for a capitated payment for the treatment of tuberculosis and requires adherence with the American Thoracic Society-Centers for Disease Control and Prevention (ATS-CDC) guidelines for the treatment of tuberculosis.

The past 3.5 years have shown this approach to be a success. From a cost standpoint, total expenditures for tuberculosis control services, including treatment, fell from about $690,000 before the contract program to about $503,000 afterward. The department pays approximately $100,000 annually to the contractor for clinical care services. The remaining $400,000 is budgeted to provide comprehensive outreach and screening to high-risk populations and surveillance and education to the private provider community. One hundred percent of patients are managed in accordance with ATS-CDC guidelines, whereas before the contract period only 79 percent of patients were managed in accordance with these guidelines and the duration of excess use of pyrazinamide and ethambutol (i.e., use of the drugs for more than 8 weeks in a patient infected with drug-susceptible organisms is considered excess use) dropped from about 16 weeks to about 1 week. Additional benefits from the contract program are that services are now available 24 hours a day from multiple sites, whereas they were available at limited times at only a single clinic before the contract, and a generally improved relationship between the private provider and the public health communities.

Keys to the success of this program included the availability of local tuberculosis expertise and an innovative and flexible health department. All agree, however, that the most important component was close communication between all the parties. The Infections Limited and health department staffs hold weekly meetings to exchange information about patients and ensure the quality of care. The cost-savings realized as a consequence of contracting direct clinical care to the private sector has enabled the health department to reinvest in primary, population-based prevention efforts without any diminution of communicable disease control services.

SOURCE: Information provided by Alan Tice and colleagues of Infections Limited and Frederico Cruz-Uribe and staff of the Pierce County Health Department.

course regimens for the treatment of latent infections. State and local programs must assume leadership roles and be responsible for the development and implementation of effective, practical tuberculin skin testing strategies based on the local epidemiological situation.

CROSSCUTTING STRATEGIES

In addition to the goal-specific effects on the evolution of tuberculosis control strategies described in the previous section, progress toward tuberculosis elimination will also require crosscutting changes in approach. These changes can be broadly grouped into three categories based on the two effects of moving toward tuberculosis elimination—declining numbers of cases and increasing competition for tuberculosis control resources—and the trend toward health care reform and reliance on managed care systems.

Response to Declining Incidence

In 1998, nearly three-quarters of all tuberculosis cases were reported in 99 metropolitan statistical areas with populations of greater than or equal to 500,000, whereas nearly half of the counties in the United States reported no cases of tuberculosis, demonstrating the increasing geographical concentration of tuberculosis in the United States. Tuberculosis elimination is dependent on tuberculosis control activities in the larger jurisdictions, including an increased emphasis on tuberculin skin testing of high-risk populations. Tuberculosis elimination, however, will not substantially influence the activities in these areas until local numbers of cases begin to decline. Instead, it is the lower-incidence jurisdictions that will first face the effects of declining numbers of cases on control strategies.

Much of the current competency of public health tuberculosis control relies on the presence of experienced personnel. As part of the normal course of work, these individuals transfer their knowledge to less experienced staff. The result is a core of competency that survives over time. One very important core of competency is the group of public health advisers employed by CDC and assigned to work in state and local health departments as direct federal assistance. Most of these individuals began their careers in public health as field workers in sexually transmitted disease, tuberculosis, or other public health programs and have worked in a variety of field and managerial positions. After a number of years of not hiring new individuals as public health advisers, the CDC Division of Tuberculosis Elimination is again recruiting and hiring new field staff. Over the years, this will help maintain a core of competency that will be invaluable.

As tuberculosis becomes less common, the system, rather than individuals within it will need to have the correct knowledge to ensure that the right steps are taken and procedures followed to control and eliminate tuberculosis. Strategies to improve this "system expertise" are described in the following sections.

Training and Technical Assistance for Providers

The most direct solution for decreased experience is increased training. To address the gap about knowledge in the care and management of patients with tuberculosis, the Strategic Plan for Tuberculosis Training and Education was recently (January 1999) released as a joint project of the National Tuberculosis Centers and the CDC Division of Tuberculosis Elimination (1999). The plan is a product of a yearlong process by leading experts in tuberculosis education and care. It provides a blueprint for building a strong, coordinated, and effective system for tuberculosis training and education and targets private-sector medical providers and related care providers (nurse practitioners, physician's assistants, etc.).

Specifically, the plan calls for a coordinated national effort to strengthen, expand, and increase access to the best ongoing educational and training opportunities in the care and management of patients with tuberculosis. This effort seeks to influence the curriculum of the nation's medical and nursing schools, strengthen training opportunities in the care and management of patients with tuberculosis for the nation's public health sector, and identify and provide training resources to strengthen private-sector and managed care management of tuberculosis.

Special training efforts should be focused on those physicians serving impoverished individuals and new arrivals to the United States, such as physicians in community health centers, migrant health centers and public hospitals, and foreign-trained physicians. Distinct educational programs are also needed for correctional institutions and the U.S. military.

Finally, the plan makes recommendations to develop linkages and partnerships to improve tuberculosis education and training, identify and catalogue training resources and programs, and improve funding to support tuberculosis training and education.

With respect to managed care, the plan outlines a number of strategies and needs that should be addressed to improve private-sector care of patients with tuberculosis. For example, by definition, "managed care" involves a third party—the health plan and its medical director—in care decisions that were previously limited to the patient and the patient's physician. This third-party involvement provides a vehicle through which new standards of care can be implemented, monitored, and when necessary, enforced. In addition, at the provider or clinician level, managed care health plans carefully review and verify through a formal process called "credentialing" the professional training and experience of each of their contracted physicians. Untoward events that might indicate substandard care (e.g., disproportionately high inpatient death rates, surgical failures, excessive return of patients to the operating room within 30 days of their surgery, high rates of malpractice claims, or surgical and diagnostic utilization rates above a regional average) are investigated and, where indicated, subjected to formal peer review by other physicians. Failure to meet a nationally accepted standard of care—especially if promulgated by the managed care organization—can result in the termination of a physician's contract with the organization and access to the health plan's members

Moreover, any such formal action can have a significant and permanent negative impact on a physician's career both through the state's physician licensing board and through the National Practitioner Data Bank, an organization established by the federal government to maintain a historical database on every physician. Hospitals, licensing organizations, insurance companies as well as governmental and military agencies, routinely review this file before establishing or renewing any formal relationship with a physician.

As the number of tuberculosis cases decline, so too will local public health and private provider experience in assessing and managing difficult tuberculosis diagnostic or treatment issues. Although informal consultation and referral systems have been established in many areas, there is a danger that these will become less used as local experience wanes and neither provider nor local tuberculosis control program will know whom to call. An example of one local health department physician's use of a "warm line" for consultation and assistance is described in the box Use of a Warm Line in a Low-Incidence Area and demonstrates the value of these systems.

Increasingly, the Internet can be used to ensure tuberculosis program staff training and competency. The recent appropriation of federal bioterrorism dollars for the creation of a Health Alert Network will result in dedicated, high-speed Internet connections, computer hardware and software to take advantage of this resource, and an increased capacity to participate in distance-based learning in most local health departments. These new tools provide a perfect opportunity to increase the "system expertise" in tuberculosis control by making the Internet a site of user-friendly training, education, and reference material.

Training and Technical Assistance for Patients and Their Significant Others

The vulnerable populations at high risk for tuberculosis infection and tuberculosis diagnosis have changed during recent years. Now, at the beginning of the 21st century, populations at high risk for tuberculosis include homeless people, substance abusers, foreign-born persons from countries with a high prevalence of tuberculosis, persons living with human immunodeficiency virus (HIV) infection or AIDS, and persons living in congregate settings, particularly correctional facilities.

The four states that report the largest number of tuberculosis cases also report the highest incidence of patients with HIV infection or AIDS. Consequently, because of the vulnerability of the immune systems of patients with HIV infection or AIDS, the number of individuals at risk for

Use of a Warm Line in a Low-Incidence Area

"We had a woman come to us recently with an extremely complex case of tuberculosis that wouldn't respond to any of the drugs physicians usually count on," says Mark Lundberg, M.D., M.P.H. "But with advice from the National Tuberculosis Warm Line, we were able to develop an effective treatment regimen, and our patient is doing very well."

Dr. Lundberg is the health officer and sole physician at the Butte County Department of Public Health in Oroville, California. Situated some 75 miles north of Sacramento, the county is largely rural, with a population of approximately 200,000.

In all, Dr. Lundberg says, it is not the kind of place where physicians expect to encounter patients with tuberculosis, let alone with patients with multidrug-resistant tuberculosis. In 1999, the county reported 4 cases of tuberculosis, in 1998 it reported 5 cases, and in 1997, the year with the largest number, it reported 13 cases.

"This disease can be a challenge for our local physicians," he says. "Although doctors do receive some training about tuberculosis in medical school, actually coming face to face with a tuberculosis patient often seems to create uncertainty in how to proceed with treatment."

Some physicians, especially those who moved into the county from larger metropolitan areas, respond by "referring the patient to the county chest clinic," he says. "But we don't have a chest clinic, nor do many other small and medium-sized counties. We simply don't have the resources to maintain such a level of specialization."

Dr. Lundberg believes that medical schools may unwittingly contribute to this problem. Since most medical schools are located in major cities, he says, it is perhaps natural for instructors to cite "refer to county chest clinic" as an appropriate course of action.

When a physician reports a case of tuberculosis to the county health department—as required by law—Dr. Lundberg offers to help the physician develop a course of treatment. The department's staff also handles the "public health" aspects of managing tuberculosis, such as conducting "directly observed therapy" to ensure that patients comply with prescribed treatments, notifying any individuals who have been exposed to the patients, and arranging shelter for patients who are homeless.

"In straightforward cases of tuberculosis, we believe that the actual treatment of patients—who often have other medical conditions—is best handled by their own physicians," says Dr. Lundberg. "We work with the physicians to provide whatever help they want. In particular, we provide them with the latest information on how to treat this disease."

When patients have multidrug-resistant tuberculosis, Dr. Lundberg takes responsibility for the medical treatment as well. In such cases, he typically seeks help from the Warm Line—in this instance, the line based at the Francis Curry Tuberculosis Center in San Francisco.

"This help has proved invaluable," Dr. Lundberg says. "Some of these cases are far more complex than any I've ever seen, and I've had little or no experience with some of the less common drugs. But the Warm Line consultants deal with tuberculosis every day. And by working together, we can develop treatment regimens tailored to my patients' needs. It's been great."

tuberculosis and HIV infection in these cities is greatly increased, which leads to the subsequent complications of treatment and adherence to multiple treatment regimens.

Although the populations at greatest risk for tuberculosis infection and tuberculosis have been identified, systematic studies for determination of intervention strategies for each of the high-risk populations have not been conducted. Studies are needed to determine how basic behavioral theories can enhance understanding for the creation of tailored interventions for each of the high-risk populations. Well-established theories such as the health belief model (Hachbaum, 1958; Rosenstock, 1990), empowerment (Rappaport, 1984), locus of control (Walton and Wallston, 1978), social learning theory (Bandura, 1977a, 1986; Perry et al., 1990), social support (Cohen and Davis, 1985; Israel, 1985), and diffusion theory (Orlandi, 1986; Orlandi et al. 1990; Rogers, 1962) can provide powerful insights for the development of educational programs targeted to each of the high-risk populations. However, these models have not been tested with the populations at high risk for tuberculosis to determine which educational strategies will be the most effective in supporting patient compliance and adherence to therapy.

The health belief model, developed in the 1950s by Hachbaum and colleagues in the Public Health Service, was conceptualized to examine the factors that motivate some people to participate in free tuberculosis screening programs compared with the factors that lead others to not participate. Through this early work, a model has evolved that individuals will take action to prevent damage to their health, screen for disease, or control a disease if the following factors are present. First, they must regard themselves as personally susceptible to a given condition; second, they believe that the condition has serious consequences; third, they believe that an action will either reduce their susceptibility or reduce the severity of the condition; and fourth, they believe that the anticipated barriers to taking action are outweighed by the benefits. This model, combined with Bandura's concept of self-efficacy (Bandura, 1977b) or with the three levels of prevention—primary, secondary, and tertiary (White et al., 1995)—can provide insights for critical behavioral change strategies.

There is very little information on the impacts that these models, such as the health belief model or concepts of self-efficacy, will have on adherence to treatment for populations at high risk for tuberculosis. As previously noted, "technology assessment and transfer in our society is a complex process involving many participants" (Centers for Disease Control, 1989, p. 24). Understanding cultural barriers to prevention, treatment, and control as well as the incentives and enablers that are most effective in enhancing compliance by specific target groups, such as increasing the return rate for reading of tuberculin skin test results among drug users at high risk of tuberculosis infection (Malotte et al., 1998), will be critical as efforts to bring about further reductions in the number of new cases are made. Research has also indicated the need to provide educational programs (Morisky et al., 1990) and to develop standardized protocols of health education to enhance the rates of adherence to treatment (Dick and Lombard, 1997).

Citing the earlier work of Addington (1979), a CDC update on tuberculosis elimination in the United States (Centers for Disease Control and Prevention, 1990) noted that noncompliance with prescribed therapy is the greatest remaining obstacle to elimination. Adherence to therapy must be tailored to patients' needs, lifestyles, social support system, and beliefs about health, and the cultural appropriateness of the educational materials must be determined. Any treatment plan should include an assessment of these factors (Centers for Disease Control and Prevention, 1994; Sumartojo, 1993). The need to understand these factors is also critical if further reductions in the numbers of new cases of *Mycobacterium tuberculosis* infection or tuberculosis are to be achieved.

Performance Measurement

The purpose of performance measurement is to explicitly assess whether progress toward the desired goals is being made and whether appropriate program activities are being undertaken to achieve those goals. It rests on the premise that what does not get measured does not get done. As staff become increasingly inexperienced, such measures will help ensure that the right information is monitored and will allow an ongoing objective assessment of whether tuberculosis control programs are performing adequately. Tuberculosis control is well suited to performance measures, as goals, strategies, and standards of practice are better delineated for tuberculosis than for many other public health programs. CDC's Tuberculosis Division already uses performance measures as an important part of its cooperative agreements with state and local programs. Current measures, however, are most complete for patient treatment, are less complete for case and contact investigations, and are least complete for tuberculin skin testing of high-risk populations. In addition, more attention is required for the development of "upstream" process measures that are better direct measures of the implementation of evidence-based best practices. The following are examples of performance indicators that would identify system delays and communication barriers:

- percentage of smear results received within 24 hours of specimen collection,

- percentage of tuberculosis cases diagnosed and percentage of patients treated as inpatients,
- percentage of tuberculosis patients requiring rehospitalization for treatment of tuberculosis or its complications,
- percentage of positive results reported within 2 weeks,
- percentage of isolates for which susceptibility data are reported (percentage for which susceptibility data are reported within 2 weeks of a positive culture),
- percentage of patients whose initial therapy is adequate on the basis of the subsequent susceptibility pattern for the patient's isolate,
- percentage of patients on therapy appropriate for the isolate's susceptibility pattern at 1 month,
- percentage of patients completing therapy,
- percentage of patients completing therapy within 9 or 12 months, and
- percentage of patients with documented conversion to negative smear and culture results.

At most three or four of these indicators should be selected for close monitoring to obtain an overall view of the program's status.

Implicit in the notion of performance measures is that the systems that collect and analyze the required information are in place, but as discussed in more detail later in this chapter, they are not. Data collection is an expensive process, and measurement of data on a more complete list of performance indicators for tuberculosis will require additional resources and carries the risk of reducing the resources available for program services. Ways to reduce this expense include the enhancement of existing systems rather than the building of new systems, whenever possible, and investment in unified systems capable of meeting local, state, and federal needs.

Investigative Guidelines, Instructions, and Templates

Increasingly, public health staff called on to investigate tuberculosis may not be experienced or may not have experience with on-site supervision. As is described in detail in Chapter 4, accessible, up-to-date, user-friendly, locally relevant, comprehensive guidelines, including step-by-step instructions, investigative algorithms, and checklists, are currently not available but could provide structure and supervision to inexperienced staff. The utility of these guidelines would be enhanced if they were integrated with or developed in tandem with tuberculosis control data and information systems.

Although improved cultural competency, incentives programs, and other measures have increased the likelihood of successful voluntary treatment, ensuring completion of antituberculosis therapy remains the public health practice situation most likely to require the invocation of coercive public health measures, including quarantine. As the numbers of tuberculosis cases decline, it will become increasingly unlikely that tuberculosis control personnel facing a situation in which legal actions may be warranted will have any firsthand experience with the risks and benefits or with the mechanics of implementing these measures. Tuberculosis regulations and laws are state specific. Synopses of these laws understandable to the nonlegally trained local public health professional, including step-by-step instructions for implementation of the necessary measures and templates of required forms and public health orders, may help ensure appropriate use and implementation of these measures.

Information Management Systems

Standardized, flexible surveillance and case-monitoring information systems that are designed to simultaneously meet local, state, and federal data needs are needed to monitor program efforts and to improve effectiveness. As a guide to ensuring complete and proper investigation, such systems become increasingly important as staff sophistication and experience become more unpredictable. Surprisingly, perhaps, such systems are not yet in place. Although in concept CDC's Tuberculosis Information Management System (TIMS) was meant to meet this need, in practice, it is a surveillance system and has failed as a case management system. Since TIMS meets primarily federal needs rather than state or local needs, adoption has been limited, at least in part due to its inability to import data (thus requiring double data entry) from existing case management systems that states and localities developed in the vacuum left by the absence of a national system. The result of the failure to implement TIMS in a timely manner has been that CDC has missed a window of opportunity to provide leadership. Instead, a number of individual tuberculosis control programs have invested considerable resources in their own (often incompatible) systems. Declining numbers of cases and less local and state experience increase the need for a more comprehensive approach designed with input from all relevant partners.

There is a pressing need for tuberculosis case reporting systems to be integrated with the systems used to report other notifiable conditions. CDC and the states are engaged in the initial development of systems for computerized electronic laboratory reporting (ELR) of notifiable diseases from public and private laboratories directly to public health departments. ELR would greatly ease some of the logistic issues around the reporting of laboratory results for tuberculosis from a regionalized system. The need for program information and management systems includes not only case reporting and management but, as importantly, contact investigation and management, monitoring of individuals receiving treatment for latent infection, and screening of high-risk populations. These systems should incorporate the data elements needed for performance measurement and a system for ongoing assessment of the preventability of local cases.

Response to Increasing Competition for Tuberculosis Control Resources

As tuberculosis elimination proceeds, the expectation (or hope) that tuberculosis control resources will remain at their current level is less than an optimum strategic approach. In the absence of daily demonstration of need, the historical example of the 1970s showed that there will be pressure to shift tuberculosis control funding to other, more visible priorities, as discussed in the previous chapter. Although the rallying cry for continued categorical funding may continue to resonate loudly in the halls of tuberculosis control programs, as a single message it may not be heard in the larger policy discussion arenas of public health departments, local city councils, or legislative assemblies. Promoting the vision of tuberculosis elimination and advocating for the necessary resources are essential parts of the response, but equally important is anticipating reductions in resources and the loss of economies of scale resulting from declining numbers of cases. Strategies to that end are described in the following sections.

Integration of Tuberculosis Control with Other, Similar Health Department Activities

The survival of tuberculosis control efforts may depend on the dissolution of aspects of tuberculosis control programs. Federal funding and much of the state and local funding for tuberculosis control are categorical; that is, the funding is specifically appropriated by the U.S. Congress or state legislatures specifically for this purpose. Advantages of this categorical funding approach include both advocacy and accountability. Legislators can clearly see the connections between funding, needs, and program activities.

Programs funded on a disease-specific basis tend to be organized and implemented on a disease-specific basis, and there is little opportunity or incentive to communicate or collaborate across program lines. As the numbers of cases decline, stable or even modestly increasing resources for tuberculosis control on a per-case basis may likely result in an absolute drop in resources. In many areas, the critical mass of funding needed to maintain tuberculosis-specific efforts might be lost. To preserve services in the face of this decreased funding, tuberculosis control programs at the state and local levels must actively search for ways to integrate activities with comparable activities performed by other categorical health department programs. Examples of such activities might include (1) merging of tuberculosis reporting and surveillance activities with HIV, sexually transmitted disease, and other infectious disease programs that rely on the same underlying notifiable disease system; (2) integrating appropriate tuberculosis case and contact investigation activities into the job descriptions of individuals performing activities related to partner notification for sexually transmitted diseases; or (3) coinvesting in activities related to outreach to high-risk populations of interest to other categorical programs, for example, programs for injection drug users and individuals with HIV, programs for urban inner-city minority populations affected by lead paint, or programs for migrant and seasonal workers affected by pesticides.

The need for these integration activities will be felt most acutely where resources are thinnest: first at the local level and then at the state level. While categorical funding is retained for tuberculosis at the national level, as the leader of tuberculosis control activities and a primary source of funding, CDC can lead the effort to ensure efficient integration at the local level. The Division of Tuberculosis Elimination can advocate and promote integration activities, develop and pilot potential approaches, and systematically identify and correct procedures or fiscal policies that are barriers to this transition. Examples of such barriers include CDC's current requirement to use reporting software that is not compatible with other CDC or state infectious disease reporting software and a time-activity reporting system for federally funded personnel that makes it cumbersome to the point of impracticality to fund the same staff from a mix of different categorical grants.

Cost Shifting to Nontuberculosis Control Budgets

As the numbers of cases of tuberculosis decrease, pressure to shift funding now allocated to tuberculosis control programs is bound to increase. Effective advocacy (as described in Chapter 7 on mobilization) may prevent the total defunding of tuberculosis control programs, as occurred in 1972 (described in Chapter 2), but the programs visited by committee members during the site visits all indicated that their program funding had decreased or was under significant pressure. A key strategy that can be used to preserve the continued availability of resources to oversee tuberculosis control is to aggressively seek appropriate opportunities to shift treatment and screening costs out of tuberculosis control budgets. State and local tuberculosis control programs can work to ensure that private insurers rather than public resources pay for diagnostic and treatment costs whenever possible. Pressure on tuberculosis control budgets could also be reduced by establishing directly observed therapy, targeted tuberculin skin test screening, and provision of treatment of latent infection as performance-based standards in the private sector. In 1993, the Medicaid Act was amended to allow states to provide Medicaid eligibility for anyone who tests tuberculin skin test positive and who also meets that state's income eligibility criteria. Medicaid funding could then be used for the diagnosis of both latent infection and active disease and the provision of treatment for both latent infection and active disease. As was pointed out by T. Westmoreland during his presentation at the second committee meeting, Medicaid has the advantage of being an entitlement: funding can expand to meet the need, and resources do not fluctuate with the interest of legislators and policy makers. Medicaid funding applies only to the poorest individuals, but these are also some of the individuals at the highest risk for tuberculosis. While many states have not included a tuberculosis option in their Medicaid program (see the Georgia and Maine site visits in Appendix C), the box, Maximizing Medicaid Reimbursement Allows Local Tuberculosis Programs to Expand Services, describes a very successful experience with the use of Medicaid funding in a county in California. Another opportunity to shift costs from the direct tuberculosis control program budget is to ensure that targeted tuberculin skin testing and treatment of latent infection are standards of practice in other publicly funded health care settings, such as correctional institutions, migrant, and community health facilities. The importance of treatment of latent infection in these facilities is addressed in the next chapter.

Regionalization

As the incidence of tuberculosis declines, economies of scale dictate that the geographical public health unit of tuberculosis control intervention in which investment of resources makes sense becomes larger. In states where the responsibility for tuberculosis control has been devolved to counties or local boards of health, regionalization will first occur among the local jurisdictions within the state. Where the state has retained sole jurisdiction, regionalization becomes relevant when economies of scale would dictate combining services among states. As a practical matter, it probably is not reasonable to expect patients to travel to regional centers for screening or treatment purposes. However, regionalization of case and contact investigation resources for the increasing number of jurisdictions with low incidences of tuberculosis is a practical way to ensure continuity of effective services. Although this might be achieved by using resources from adjacent local jurisdictions, in many cases the coordination role will fall to the state tuberculosis control program in the form of personnel with specific job responsibilities to serve as ad hoc providers of services, including case and contact investigations and perhaps administration of directly observed therapy. Similar regionalization of services will also be required among states. CDC can promote this regionalization through pilot programs that could be funded within cooperative agreements with the states.

The issue of regionalization of laboratory services may already be an issue for many areas. As noted in the consultant's report in Appendix D, 10 to 15 specimens a week need to be examined to maintain proficiency in a Level I tuberculosis laboratory. A Level I laboratory prepares and examines smears only. Laboratories that provide more sophisticated services, including culture, species determination, and susceptibility testing should be processing at least 25 isolates per week to maintain proficiency, according to the consultant's report. It is likely that many state laboratories already have workloads too small to maintain proficiency, and again, CDC could promote regionalization through pilot programs.

CDC may also be able to promote regionalization if it maintains personnel with the expertise for backup during outbreak situations and for complex investigations. Public health advisers, Epidemic Intelligence Service officers and staff epidemiologists and clinical field staff employed by the Division of Tuberculosis Elimination have successfully supplied this type of expertise in the past. If this capability is not maintained within CDC, it is difficult to identify where it should be obtained when needed.

Capacity Measures

As the numbers of cases of tuberculosis decline, the perceived need for active tuberculosis control programs will become less apparent. Policy makers will lose touch with the issue and health departments may be unsure or unable to effectively articulate their specific resource requirements. Public health capacity measures (measures of the system's "ability to provide specific services, such as clinical screening or disease surveillance, made possible by the maintenance of the basic infrastructure of the public health system, as well as specific program resources") provide part of the answer. For example, adherence to capacity measures for case investigation will help ensure that a jurisdiction with no cases of tuberculosis for several years will have the required competency when the next case arises. In general, such measures are not available, and better definition and promotion of expert-generated, nationally accepted measures of

Maximizing Medicaid Reimbursement Allows
Local Tuberculosis Programs to Expand Services:
A Success Story in California

In 1994, the California legislature enacted legislation that created the California Medicasi (Medi-Cal) Tuberculosis (MCTB) program benefit. Persons with known or suspected tuberculosis infection or disease who cannot qualify for full-scope Medi-Cal benefits but who meet less stringent criteria that are federally defined, can qualify as beneficiaries for the MCTB program.

The California Department of Health Services developed the MCTB program to provide a new funding source for local health jurisdiction (LHJ) tuberculosis programs to cover costs that would otherwise be incurred by categorical local, state, and federal dollars. For those persons who qualify only for the tuberculosis treatment benefit, the program covers outpatient tuberculosis treatment services including directly observed therapy (DOT) and directly observed preventive therapy (DOPT) at $19.23 per encounter. An LHJ can also receive reimbursement for DOT and DOPT provided to full Medi-Cal beneficiaries. A crucial first step, however, is the ability of the tuberculosis program to enroll beneficiaries.

Tuberculosis programs have encountered several challenges to identifying potential beneficiaries and enrolling them in MCTB. Foreign-born clients often fear that enrollment in the program will prevent them from obtaining citizenship. Other challenges include the absence of a well-established working relationship between the tuberculosis control program and the Department of Social Services or decentralized tuberculosis care systems with multiple clinics necessitating screening and enrollment at numerous sites.

Santa Clara County, through a partnership of its Tuberculosis Program and Ambulatory Care Tuberculosis Clinic, has been the most successful of the California tuberculosis control programs. In 1998, Santa Clara County reported 251 cases of tuberculosis; 87.6 percent were foreign-born Asians. Each year Santa Clara County evaluates approximately 400 new immigrants suspected of contracting tuberculosis overseas (B notification). About 25 percent of the tuberculosis clinic patients qualify for full Medi-Cal benefits. An additional approximately 14 percent of patients are enrolled in the MCTB program. The annual budget for the tuberculosis clinic is $1.4 million.

the capacities of effective tuberculosis control programs are needed. These measures, linked to accountability and funding, can serve as a useful adjunct to process and outcome performance measures to ensure continued competency to respond to increasingly uncommon events.

Response to Managed Care

The percentage of individuals with tuberculosis who receive care in the private sector is likely to grow, as Medicaid and Medicare recipients are increasingly being enrolled in the health plans of private for-profit insurance companies and managed care organizations. In 1997, the last

For fiscal year 1999–2000 Santa Clara County is estimating $300,000 in revenue to the tuberculosis clinic from Medi-Cal reimbursements for outpatient tuberculosis testing and treatment services, including DOT-DOPT. Significant savings are gained through direct billing of Medi-Cal for medications and laboratory services. Approximately $100,000 in additional income is projected through the Health Care Finance Administration's Medi-Cal Administrative Services reimbursement.

Santa Clara County's success is due to several factors: two full-time financial counselors in the tuberculosis clinic, a dedicated tuberculosis clinic, good marketing skills that result in a win–win approach that both benefits patients and enhances clinical services, development of a strong relationship with the Department of Social Services, and perseverance.

The financial counselors play a key role. At the first visit each patient is interviewed regarding his or her financial status. Although some credibility is gained because they are immigrants themselves, the counselors' effectiveness results largely from their knowledgeable, culturally sensitive approach. Patients are told that they may be eligible for a variety of programs that will cover the cost of their care. It is clearly explained why enrollment will not prevent the granting of citizenship, and the benefits of coverage, even for Nontuberculosis conditions, are emphasized. Patients are assisted with their applications and are told to bring to the counselors any bills that they receive while waiting for approval for participation in the program. It is also emphasized that no one will be denied services on the basis of an ability to pay, whether or not they qualify for Medi-Cal. The patients appreciate the concern and assistance with their financial problems.

In the face of level state and federal categorical funding for tuberculosis, the MCTB program has enabled Santa Clara County to expand and improve tuberculosis treatment services. MCTB program revenues are paying for the financial counselors and have helped the tuberculosis program upgrade several positions.

SOURCE: Karen Lee Smith, MD, MPH, and Elizabeth Kinoshita, PHN, Santa Clara County Tuberculosis Control Program, and Deborah Tabor, RN, Tuberculosis Branch, California Department of Health Services.

year for which data are available, more than 14 percent of Medicare patients and 52 percent of Medicaid patients were in some type of managed care program. Moreover, academic medical centers, public hospitals, veteran's facilities, and community and migrant health centers, once closely cooperative with health departments are also increasingly functioning as private providers, competing for patient populations and billing on a fee-for-service basis.

Another health sector reform with the potential to significantly affect tuberculosis control is the growing trend toward privatization by local health departments. Privatization, which consists of outsourcing or contracting with private for-profit or not-for-profit organizations to provide services and care formerly provided directly by the health department, is being widely adopted by local health departments in response to reductions in public funding by federal, state, and local governments (Bialek and Chaulk, 1999).

Unless these reforms, however, are addressed in a clear, forthright, and consistent manner throughout the country, they could pose a real threat to the elimination of tuberculosis in the United States. For example, local health departments are the focal point for tuberculosis control efforts across the United States. Many local health departments use Medicaid dollars to cross-subsidize wraparound services for more comprehensive management of communicable diseases such as tuberculosis. Moving the responsibility for the care of patients who are recipients of public aid (e.g., Medicaid or Medicare patients) and the concomitant funds for care for those patients to the private sector will make the previously available financial resources inaccessible to public health agencies. The problems associated with an inadequately planned privatization of tuberculosis treatment services were clearly observed in a series of failed pilot projects in Pennsylvania (Lopez, 1999).

At the same time, according to a recent national analysis, state Medicaid managed care contracts are virtually devoid of language delineating the management of tuberculosis patients. Thus, most managed care organizations that care for Medicaid patients are not bound by any standard of care in the treatment of tuberculosis. Since traditional private sector health care models are ill equipped to provide the comprehensive public health services necessary for effective tuberculosis control, these shifts in patients and resources could jeopardize this public health effort.

Opportunities

On the other hand, managed care and privatization present, at least in theory, opportunities to redefine and strengthen the respective roles of local health departments and private-sector health care organizations in support of a national tuberculosis control and elimination effort. This is attainable if population-based approaches to care are addressed by managed care organizations and other organizations contracting with state or local health departments. The emergence of managed care and the evolution of its organizational and fiscal technologies present additional opportunities for strengthening tuberculosis control efforts. These opportunities include an emphasis on identifiable points of accountability for client outcomes; varying levels of risk sharing among providers, clients, and managed care organizations; the use of pooled resources across systems; a prevention-focused orientation; ongoing outcome-oriented quality assurance activities; and accreditation requirements.

Moreover, because of the combined advent of managed care and privatization, many health departments are no longer simply providers of care. Today, many local health departments and virtually all state Medicaid programs are purchasers of care. This newfound role provides them a mechanism by which they can balance their fiscal pressures with their public health obligations.

For example, as purchasers, these public organizations can specify the desired relationships, products, and outcomes through their contractual processes. As in the example cited earlier in a box in this chapter describing the experience in Pierce County, Washington, contracts can set performance standards and identify necessary organizational capacities, technical expertise, provider competencies, and the laboratory quality control necessary for private-sector organizations to successfully undertake the treatment and management of tuberculosis patients. Contracts can also can be used to align public and private stakeholders so that tuberculosis control is properly coordinated among these partners and their participating provider and laboratory networks. In an effort to improve the contract process, CDC staff have developed model contract language that can be adopted for managed care or privatization purposes (Miller et al., 1998). However, these model contracts have not been field tested.

Quality Assurance

Initially adopted as a tool to counter ever rising health care costs, the managed care system is increasingly focusing on improved health outcomes. This focus on quality reflects, in part, recognition that costs and quality are intertwined. Thus, a short-term saving, only to be followed by even worse and more costly-to-treat outcomes, is a poor trade-off. The current climate of reform in health care provides several opportunities to improve and sustain quality care for tuberculosis patients.

First, the National Committee on Quality Assurance (NCQA), a body whose board includes representatives from major employer and consumer groups, has developed criteria that can be used to monitor quality in the delivery of health care. The board has strongly endorsed a formal NCQA accreditation process that involves defined standards, measures of achievement, and quality-of-care audits. Failure to achieve NCQA accreditation can adversely affect a managed care organization's ability to successfully compete for employer group insurance contracts.

NCQA's board has adopted a wide array of nationally established preventive health standards (e.g., rates of immunizations and rates of ophthalmologic screening for diabetic retinopathy) and has recently moved into establishing standards of treatment (e.g., treatment with beta-blocking agents after a myocardial infarction). Health plans seeking to acquire or maintain NCQA accreditation are expected to measure and meet these standards. These standards, as well as other key components of managed care programs—from provider clinical responsibilities and duties, to economic incentives and patient and provider risk sharing, access to specialists, patient benefits, and all other aspects of service and financing—are based on legally binding contracts between the health plan and selected physician and institutional providers.

In addition, the health plan seeks discounts in physician and institutional payments in exchange for clinical access to its members, but only for those physicians who agree to participate in the health plan and comply with its contract obligations. Through these processes, the health plan becomes responsible for the quality of care provided to its members by those physicians contracted into the plan's provider network. The accreditation body for hospitals and other institutional health providers, the Joint Commission on Accreditation of Healthcare Organizations, is also incorporating patient care and service delivery standards into its accreditation program.

CDC, working in conjunction with state and local health departments, professional societies, and voluntary, nongovernmental organizations, has established national standards of care for tuberculosis. These standards are designed to achieve the maximum rate of cure. Not only are these standards important to the individual but they also simultaneously protect the members of the managed care organizations. If NCQA were encouraged to incorporate these standards into its quality assurance program, contracts between state Medicaid agencies and managed care organizations could also incorporate these standards as a condition of contract compliance.

Laboratory Performance Standards and Case Reporting Requirements

Access to quality microbiological services and prompt case finding and reporting are essential to the successful management of tuberculosis. A more complete discussion of the laboratory is contained in the consultant's report included in Appendix D. Several avenues that will ensure access to quality tuberculosis laboratory services and case reporting are discussed here.

As a requirement to do business within a state, commercial health plans must obtain approval of that state's division of insurance and department of health or social welfare, depending upon the state. As a result, state health departments have an administrative opportunity to influence the patient care requirements that must be met by all insurance organizations and health plans through their own regulations or through the development of a working relationship with the state division of insurance or other administrative department.

It is important that health maintenance organizations, private health plans, and contracted providers, as third parties directly involved in the overall care of their member populations, be required to promptly report all cases of tuberculosis to the state health department. Such a requirement is vital to any national effort to eliminate tuberculosis, because to minimize their laboratory expenses, many managed care organizations contract with national vendors for centralized laboratory services. Cultures for tuberculosis are often included in such contracts, with the result that positive cultures may be identified in locations out-of-state and thus may be beyond the direct surveillance powers of the health department in the state where the case of tuberculosis originated.

Early case identification followed by prompt case-contact evaluation and treatment of latent infection has been demonstrated to be the most effective means of minimizing the incidence of new cases of tuberculosis. Therefore, in the absence of state requirements for case reporting, national legislation may be necessary to ensure that all positive tuberculosis cultures are reported to the official health agency in the respective jurisdiction. Even when the state's health department lacks independent authority, and cooperation with the Division of Insurance has not developed, state or local boards of health usually have legislatively authorized power to establish rules and regulations that require that the state's physicians and hospital providers adhere to specific behavior or treatment standards. This has been successfully accomplished in Colorado and other states where specific statewide treatment standards require the implementation of directly observed therapy for all tuberculosis patients, unless an exemption is granted from the Department of Health. ERISA plans, which are privately funded and federally regulated, may be more difficult to influence, but a court decision in New York supports the position that state regulations for public health purposes can be extended to ERISA plans.

Standards of Care in Case Management

There is now clear and compelling evidence, both within the United States and internationally, that a patient-centered approach to care that uses directly observed therapy is a clinically appropriate and cost-effective strategy for the treatment of active tuberculosis (Bayer and Wilkinson, 1995). This approach produces the highest treatment completion rates because the patient is given a meaningful opportunity to work with the case management team in the design and implementation of how therapy can best be provided (Figure 3-1). To maximize treatment completion,

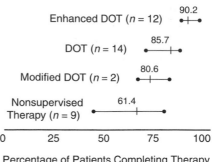

FIGURE 3-1 Range and median treatment completion rates, by treatment intervention, for pulmonary tuberculosis reported in 27 studies. DOT, directly observed therapy; n, number of studies. SOURCE: Chaulk and Kazandjian (1998). Reprinted with permission

patient-centered programs identify and use a broad range of enablers and incentives based on the individual needs and circumstances of that particular patient. These include treatment at settings convenient for the patient (workplace, home, school); the provision of relevant social and economic enablers and incentives such as food, clothing, books, stipends, transportation, treatment contracts, bilingual staff, and reminder systems; and culturally appropriate outreach and tracking for missed appointments (Chan et al., 1994; Chaulk and Kazandjian, 1998; Chaulk et al., 1995; El-Sadr et al., 1996; Kan et al., 1985; Manalo et al., 1990; Miles and Maat, 1984; Pozsik et al., 1993; Schluger et al., 1995; Sukrakanchana-Trikham et al., 1992; Werhane et al., 1989; Westaway et al., 1991; Wilkinson, 1994). Moreover, these programs are sometimes supplemented with substance abuse treatment and counseling (Chaulk et al., 1995; Schluger et al., 1995; Werhane et al., 1989), housing for homeless patients (during therapy) (Chaulk et al., 1995), comprehensive case management, and referral for other medical and social services as indicated (Chan et al., 1994; El-Sadr et al., 1996; Werhane et al., 1989). Importantly, these patient-centered approaches coupled with directly observed therapy and other aspects of case supervision have been shown to be highly effective across a range of geographical and socioeconomic settings, producing treatment completion rates in excess of 90 percent (Bayer et al., 1998). The provision of incentives without directly observed therapy produces much lower completion rates (Armstrong and Pringle, 1984; Caminero et al., 1996; Cohn et al., 1990; Cowie and Brink, 1990; Dutt et al., 1984; Hong Kong Chest Service/British Medical Research Council, 1984; Jin et al., 1993; Menzies et al., 1993; Ormerod et al., 1991; Samuel, 1976; Snider et al., 1998; Valeza and McCougall, 1990; Van der Werf et al., 1990; Wolde et al., 1992). Similarly, while legal orders mandate completion of treatment, they do not replace patient-centered approaches to care, which have been successful without the use of legal orders (Pozsik et al., 1993).

Failure to complete a course of recommended therapy can have several adverse outcomes, including the development of drug-resistant disease. The reasons for these failures are multifactorial (Chaulk and Kazandjian, 1998). They may include failure of the patient to take all or part of his or her medications. Studies have clearly documented that 30 to 35 percent of self-administered medications are not taken. Directly observed therapy diminishes this possibility, as long as the third party observing the ingestion of medication (nurse, doctor, or other health care worker) actually watches to confirm that each dose is taken. Other reasons may be either provider or system related. For example, providers may fail to prescribe an appropriate treatment regimen or may inappropriately add drugs to a regimen. The system of care may not address the cultural or lifestyle needs of the patient. Programs that assess and address all of the potential obstacles to treatment delivery (patient as well as system related) are the most successful (Chaulk and Kazandjian, 1998). Tuberculosis treatment in managed care or any private setting must be viewed in this context.

Good contract terms for standards of care and quality of care for both managed care and private-sector arrangements define the respective roles of public- and private-sector stakeholders in ensuring that therapy is supervised or closely monitored. Such arrangements should be designed around the respective strengths of these public and private entities and are a key part of the contracts discussed earlier for the city of Tacoma and for Pierce County in Washington State. In addition, state action can further strengthen this arrangement. Colorado's Department of Health has recently established specific statewide treatment standards that require the implementation of directly observed therapy for all patients identified as having active tuberculosis unless an exemption is obtained from the Department of Health. In situations where directly observed therapy can not be used, fixed-dose drug combinations (containing both isoniazid and rifampin) should be used to reduce the risk of developing resistance to either drug.

Centralized Data Management

Centralized management information systems are becoming increasingly common tools of managed care organizations. An adequate management information system capacity can be used to improve the quality of care for patients with tuberculosis by profiling providers, tracking laboratory services and pharmacological regimens, especially when they are

Baltimore City Case Study

For more than 22 years, the Baltimore City Health Department's Tuberculosis Control Program has used directly observed therapy (DOT) for the treatment of patients with pulmonary tuberculosis. The Baltimore City Health Department launched its DOT program in 1978 by targeting tuberculosis patients who were homeless, unemployed, alcoholics, or substance abusers. DOT was provided under nursing supervision at the city's tuberculosis Chest Clinics. In 1982, DOT was brought into the community for all tuberculosis patients. Nurses provided supervised therapy at the patient's home, workplace, or school. Between 1978 and 1995, the incidence of tuberculosis declined 62 percent whereas Baltimore's ranking for tuberculosis (typically ranked highest between 1965 and 1978) fell from 2nd in 1978 to 28th by 1992.

The hallmark of this program has been a patient-centered approach that uses nurse outreach to provide care and ongoing evaluation of the patient throughout the course of the patient's therapy.

In addition to the dramatic decline in the rate of tuberculosis following implementation of DOT, even during the resurgence years of 1985 to 1992, other program benchmarks indicate other successes. The rate of sputum conversion by 3 months of therapy is twofold higher for patients managed with DOT compared to private-sector patients who receive self-administered therapy. Multidrug resistance has essentially been eliminated (less that 0.05 percent of all cases), therapy completion rates are greater than 95 percent by 12 months of therapy, and the rate of mortality during therapy is fourfold lower for patients managed with DOT than for private-sector patients. These benchmarks apply to AIDS patients as well when they are managed with DOT. Additional research suggests that Baltimore's DOT program is cost-effective compared to self-administered therapy, and the reduction in the number of expected cases under this program has generated savings that are at least double the actual operating costs of this program.

SOURCE: Data from P. Chaulk and the Baltimore City Health Department.

coordinated with the reporting and surveillance practices of local health departments.

The contract process can establish minimum performance standards regarding management information system performance that a managed care organization's provider network must adhere to as part of its participation in the managed care organization's plan. Simple sharing of provider inpatient and outpatient care practices on a geographical basis, along with comparing provider comparisons with national practice guidelines, has proved to be a powerful tool for improving quality of patient care.

Community Health Centers

The successful control and eventual elimination of tuberculosis in the United States will rest upon the efforts derived from strategic public–private partnerships that can leverage the resources and public will necessary to achieve these goals. In health care, the nation's oldest safety net is made up of publicly funded general hospitals and urban, rural, and migrant health centers.

Community health centers are the entry point to the U.S. health care system for more than 10 million people (Davis et al., 1999). Most community health center clients are either uninsured (41 percent) or on Medicaid (33 percent). More importantly, community health centers serve those people most at risk for tuberculosis. In 1996, community health centers provided health care to more than 450,000 homeless children and adults and another 500,000 seasonal and migrant workers. In addition, 65 percent of all community health center clients are ethnic minorities.

Although traditionally funded with governmental monies, these institutions—public hospitals, community health center clinics, neighborhood health centers, clinics for refugees and immigrants, and their physicians—provide care under the same principles that the private sector of medicine uses. However, the progressive transfer of Medicaid patients into private insurance plans has required these institutions to seek contracts with managed care organizations to ensure ongoing funding sources. As a result, the discounted payments offered by managed care organizations can produce substantial revenue losses, straining already overburdened and overcrowded health care systems.

Nonetheless, this change offers an additional opportunity to establish and enforce nationwide standards of care for patients with tuberculosis. Partnerships between these providers that serve the most vulnerable populations, local health departments, and managed care organizations would result in improved access to tuberculosis services in the primary care setting. Such partnerships could also involve the wide range of other organizations and providers that provide primary care to those most at risk of developing tuberculosis. Such organizations include health and resettlement centers for political refugees and new immigrants, organizations that serve populations on both sides of the United States-Mexico border, programs that serve homeless people, substance abuse treatment centers, programs that serve people with HIV infection and AIDS, the child welfare system, and corrections systems.

CDC cooperative grants have been most effective in redirecting the tuberculosis program efforts of health departments. Similar initiatives by federal agencies that support the services of the multiple components of the safety net could have a significant and long-term nationwide impact on the treatment, prevention, and control of tuberculosis.

CONCLUSION

Although the goals and functions of tuberculosis control programs are constant, as the United States moves toward tuberculosis elimination, their implementation will require changes in strategies and activities. The directions of change described in this initial assessment can and should evolve over time.

The expertise present in federal, state, and local programs should be brought to bear on this process. This same expertise and leadership must also increasingly serve both as a credible voice of advocacy for the vision of tuberculosis elimination and as an agent for change in tuberculosis control activities. In some respects, the latter task may be the most difficult one. Bureaucracies, including public health bureaucracies, are not known for their capacity to change quickly. The skills required for the increased emphasis on the assurance of quality tuberculosis services and care and screening of high-risk populations may not match the existing workforce skills of tuberculosis program staff. Careful attention must be paid to ensuring that tuberculosis control programs become what they need to be rather than maintained as they have been.

REFERENCES

Addington WW. 1979. Patient compliance: The most serious remaining problem in the control of tuberculosis in the United States. *Chest* 76(Suppl):741–743.

American Thoracic Society and Centers for Disease Control and Prevention. 2000. Targeted tuberculin testing and treatment of latent infection. *Am J Respir Crit Care Med* 161: 5221–5247.

Armstrong RH, and Pringle D. 1984. Compliance with anti-tuberculosis chemotherapy in Harare City. *Cent Afr J Med* 30:144–148.

Bandura A. 1977a. *Social Learning Theory*. Englewood Cliffs, NJ: Prentice-Hall.

Bandura A. 1977b. Self-efficacy: Toward a unifying theory of behavior change. *Psychol Rev* 84:191–215.

Bandura A. 1986. *Social Foundations of Thought and Action*. Englewood Cliffs, NJ: Prentice-Hall.

Bayer R, Stayton C, Desvarieux MD, et al., 1998. Directly observed therapy and treatment completion for tuberculosis in the United States: Is universal supervised therapy necessary? *Am J Public Health* 88:1052–1058.

Bayer R, and Wilkinson D. 1995. Directly observed therapy for tuberculosis: History of an idea. *Lancet* 345:1545–1548.

Bialek R, and Chaulk CP. 1999. *Privatization and Public Health: A Study of in initiatives and early lessons learned*. Washington, DC: Public Health Foundation.

Caminero JA, Pavon JM, de Castro FR, et al. 1996. Evaluation of a directly observed 6-month fully intermittent treatment regimen for tuberculosis in patients suspected of poor compliance. *Thorax* 51:1130–1133.

Centers for Disease Control and Prevention. 1989. A strategic plan for the elimination of tuberculosis in the United States. *MMWR* 38:1–23.

Centers for Disease Control and Prevention. 1990. Update: Tuberculosis elimination— United States. *MMWR* 39:153–156.

Centers for Disease Control and Prevention. 1994. Improving patient adherence to tuberculosis treatment. Atlanta: CDC.

Chan SL, Wong PC, and Tam CM. 1994. 4-,5- and 6-Month regimens containing isoniazid, rifampicin, pyrazinamide and streptomycin for treatment of pulmonary tuberculosis under program conditions in Hong Kong. *Tubercle Lung Dis* 75:245–250.

Chaulk CP, and Kazandjian VA. 1998. Directly observed therapy for treatment completion of tuberculosis. Consensus statement of the Public Health Tuberculosis guidelines Panel. *JAMA* 279:943–948.

Chaulk CP, Moore-Rice K, Rizzo R, and Chaisson RE. 1995. Eleven years of community-based directly observe therapy for tuberculosis. *JAMA* 274:945–951.

Cohen S, and Davis SL. Eds. 1985. *Social Support and Health.* Orlando, FL: Academic Press.

Cohn DL, Catlin BJ, Peterson KL, Judson FN, and Sbarbaro JA. 1990. A 62-dose, 6-month therapy for pulmonary and extra-pulmonary tuberculosis: A twice-weekly, directly observed, and cost-effective regimen. *Ann Intern Med* 112:407–415.

Cowie RL, and Brink BA. 1990. Short-course chemotherapy for pulmonary tuberculosis with a rifampicin-isoniazid-pyrazinamide combination tablet. *S Afr Med J* 77:390–391.

Davis K, Collins KS, and Hall A. 1999. Community Health Centers in a Changing U.S. Health Care System. Policy Brief. New York: The Commonwealth Fund.

Dick J, and Lombard JD. 1997. Shared vision—A health education project designed to enhance adherence to anti-tuberculosis treatment. *Int J Tuberc Lung Dis* 1(2):181–186.

Dutt AK, Moers D, and Stead WW. 1984. Short-course chemotherapy for tuberculosis with mainly twice-weekly isoniazid and rifampin: Community physicians' seven-year experience with mainly outpatients. *Am J Med* 77:233–242.

El-Sadr W, Medard F, and Barthaud V. 1996. Directly observed therapy for tuberculosis: The Harlem Hospital experience, 1993. *Am J Public Health* 86:1146–1149.

Hachbaum GM. 1958. *Public Participation in Medical Screening Programs: A Sociopsychological Study.* Bethesda, MD: U.S. Public Health Service.

Hong Kong Chest Service/British Medical Research Council. 1984. Study of a fully supervised programme of chemotherapy for pulmonary tuberculosis given once weekly in the continuation phase in the rural areas of Hong Kong. *Tubercle* 65:5–15.

Institute of Medicine. 1988. *The Future of Public Health.* Washington, DC: National Academy Press.

Israel B. 1985. Social networks and social support: Implications for natural helper and community level intervention. *Health Educ Q* 12:66–80.

Jin BW, Kim SC, Mori T, and Shimao T. 1993. The impact of intensified supervisory activities on tuberculosis treatment. *Tubercle Lung Dis* 74:267–272.

Kan G, Zhang L, Wu J, and Ma Z. 1985. Supervised intermittent chemotherapy for pulmonary in a rural area of China. *Tubercule* 66:1–7.

Lopez S. 1999. Critics blast attempt to privatize health centers in Pennsylvania. *State Health Watch Newsl* 6(4):1, 5–6.

Malotte CK, Rhodes F, and Mais KE. 1998. Tuberculosis screening and compliance with return for skin test reading among active drug users. *Am J Public Health* 88:792–796.

Manalo F, Tan F, Sbarbaro JA, and Iseman MD. 1990. Community-based short-course treatment of pulmonary tuberculosis in a developing nation: Initial report of an eight-month, largely intermittent regimen in a population with a high prevalence of drug resistance. *Am Rev Respir Dis* 142:1301–1305.

Menzies R, Rocher I, and Vissandjee B. 1993. Factors associated with compliance in treatment of tuberculosis. *Tubercl Lung Dis* 74:32–37.

Miles SH, and Maat RB. 1984. A successful supervised outpatient short-course tuberculosis treatment program in an open refugee camp on the Thai-Cambodian border. *Am Rev Respir Dis* 130:827–830.

Miller B, Rosenbaum S, Strange PV, Solomon SL, and Castro KG. 1998. Tuberculosis control in a changing health care system: Model contract specifications for managed care organizations. *Clin Infect Dis* 27(4):677–686.

Morisky DE, Malotte CK, Choi P, et al. 1990. A patient education program to improve adherence rates with antituberculosis drug regimes. *Health Educ Q* 17:253–267.

Orlandi MA. 1986. The diffusion and adoption of worksite health promotion innovations: An analysis of the barriers. *Prev Med* 15:522–536.

Orlandi MA, Landers KC, Weston R, et al. 1990. Diffusion of health promotion innovations. In: *Health Behavior and Health Education* (K Glanz, FM Lewis, and BK Rimer, eds.). San Francisco: Jossey-Bass.

Ormerod LP, McCarthy O, Rudd RM, and Horsfield N. 1991. Short-course chemotherapy for pulmonary tuberculosis. *Respir Med* 85:291–294.

Perry CL, Baranowski T, and Parcel GS. 1990. How individuals, environments, and health behavior interact: Social learning theory. In: *Health Behavior and Health Education* (K Glanz, FM Lewis, and BK Rimer, eds.). San Francisco: Jossey-Bass.

Pozsik C, Kinney J, Breeden D, Nivin B, and Davis T. 1993. Approaches to improving adherence to antituberculosis therapy—South Carolina and New York, 1986–1992. *MMWR* 42:74–75, 81.

Rappaport J. 1984. Studies in empowerment: Introduction to the issue. *Prev Hum Services* 3:1–7.

Rogers EM. 1962. *Diffusion of Innovations*, 3rd ed. New York: Free Press.

Rosenstock IM. 1990. The Health Belief Model. In: *Health Behavior and Health Education* (K Glanz, FM Lewis, and BK Rimer, eds.). San Francisco: Jossey-Bass.

Samuel GER. 1976. Use of discriminate analysis for improving treatment completion in district tuberculosis programme. *Indian J Public Health* 20:21–24.

Sbarbaro JA. 1970. The public health tuberculosis clinic—Its place in comprehensive health care. *Am Rev Respir Dis* 101:463–465.

Schluger N, Ciotoli C, Cohen D, Johnson H, and Rom WN. 1995. Comprehensive tuberculosis control for patients at high risk of noncompliance. *Am J Respir Crit Care Med* 151:1486–1490.

Snider DD, Long MW, Cross FS, and Farer LS. 1984. Six-month isoniazid-rifampin therapy for pulmonary tuberculosis: Report of a United States Public Health Service cooperative trial. *Am Rev Respir Dis* 129:573–579.

Sukrakanchana-Trikham P, Puechal X, Rigal J, and Rieder HL. 1992. Ten-year assessment of treatment outcome among Cambodian refugees with sputum smear-positive tuberculosis in Khao-1-Dang, Thailand. *Tubercle Lung Dis* 73:384–387.

Sumartojo E. 1993. When tuberculosis treatment fails: A social behavioral account of patient adherence. *Am Rev Respir Dis* 147:1311–1320.

Valeza FS, and McCougall AC. 1990. Blister calendar packs for treatment of tuberculosis. *Lancet* 335:473.

Van der Werf TS, Dade GK, and Van der Mark TW. 1990. Patient compliance with tuberculosis treatment in Ghana: Factors influencing adherence to therapy in a rural service programme. *Tubercule* 71:247–252.

Walton KS, and Wallston BS. 1978. Locus of control and health. *Health Educ Monogr* 6:107–117.

Werhane MJ, Snukst-Torbeck G, and Schraufnagel DE. 1989. The tuberculosis clinic. *Chest* 96:815–818.

White GL, Henthorne BH, Barnes SE, and Segarra JT. 1995. Tuberculosis: A health education imperative returns. *J Comm Health* 20:29–57.

Wolde K, Lema E, Roscigno G, and Abdi A. 1992. Fixed dose combination short course chemotherapy in the treatment of pulmonary tuberculosis. *Ethiop Med J* 30:63–68.

4

Advancing Toward Elimination

Once the control of tuberculosis is ensured through the treatment of active cases of tuberculosis, the next step in tuberculosis control is to focus on the prevention of new cases. The relatively long interval between infection with *Mycobacterium tuberculosis* and the onset of disease creates an opportunity to intervene and prevent disease by treating those with latent infection. Also, as the risk of infection declines, more cases will be the result of reactivation of infection acquired many years earlier. Increasing efforts at prevention can accelerate the decline in the number of cases of tuberculosis, maintain momentum and interest in tuberculosis control programs, and act as preparation for a final push to elimination. This chapter provides an overview of the principles of prevention through treatment of latent infection and proposes strategies for use of this approach with defined populations including foreign-born individuals, especially recent arrivals, from countries with high rates of tuberculosis, inmates of correctional facilities, infected contacts of individuals with infectious tuberculosis, and other high-risk groups that are defined locally. The committee recognizes that many of the strategies described in this chapter will require significant changes and increases in resources at all levels of tuberculosis control but is convinced of the importance of accelerating efforts for the prevention of tuberculosis.

RECOMMENDATIONS

Recommendation 4.1 To limit the spread of tuberculosis from infec-

tious patients to their contacts, the committee recommends that more effective methodologies for the identification of persons with recently acquired tuberculosis infection, especially persons exposed to patients with new cases of tuberculosis, be developed and efforts be increased to evaluate appropriately and treat latent infection in all persons who meet the criteria for treatment for such infections.

Recommendation 4.2 To prevent the development of tuberculosis among individuals with latent tuberculosis infection, the committee recommends that

• Tuberculin skin testing be required as part of the medical evaluation for immigrant visa applicants from countries with high rates of tuberculosis, a Class B4 immigration waiver designation be created for persons with normal chest radiographs and positive tuberculin skin tests, and all tuberculin-positive Class B immigrants be required to undergo an evaluation for tuberculosis and, when indicated, complete an approved course of treatment for latent infection before receiving a permanent residency card ("green card"). Implementation should be in a stepwise fashion and pilot programs should evaluate and assess costs.

• Tuberculin testing be required of all inmates of correctional facilities and completion of an approved course of treatment, when indicated, be required, with referral to the appropriate public health agency for all inmates released before completion of treatment.

• Programs of targeted tuberculin skin testing and treatment of latent infection be increased for high-incidence groups, such as HIV-infected individuals, undocumented immigrants, homeless individuals, and intravenous drug abusers, as determined by local epidemiological circumstances.

BACKGROUND AND INTRODUCTION

The recent success of tuberculosis control efforts indicates that, given adequate resources, the traditional control program that focuses on the treatment of active tuberculosis is once again functioning effectively and that a steady decline in cases should be expected. However, to make significant progress toward the elimination of tuberculosis in the United States, efforts to prevent cases from occurring must be amplified. Without an effective vaccine for the prevention of pulmonary tuberculosis, the most effective means of preventing new cases is to take advantage of the relatively long period between infection and the development of active disease by treating individuals with latent infection to reduce the risk of disease. The Advisory Council for the Elimination of Tuberculosis (ACET) included expanded targeted testing and treatment of latent infection among the highest-priority activities for tuberculosis control programs (CDC, 1999). Recently published guidelines from the Centers for Disease Control and Prevention (CDC) and the American Thoracic Society will provide a framework for increased attention to targeted screening and will recommend new regimens for the treatment of tuberculosis infection (American Thoracic Society and CDC, 2000). As recommended by the guidelines and by ACET, local epidemiological conditions will guide the testing effort, but increased national attention will be needed in three areas. First, as noted in Chapter 2, tuberculosis among foreign-born individuals accounts for an increasing proportion of U.S. tuberculosis cases, and slightly more than half of these cases occur within the first 5 years of the arrival of foreign-born individuals in the United States. Targeted tuberculin skin testing of newly arrived immigrants before arrival in the United States with adequate treatment for those with latent infection once they arrive could prevent a significant number of cases. Second, an outbreak of tuberculosis associated with a prison led to the recognition of the resurgence of tuberculosis in the United States, and screening for infection and treatment of latent infection should be mandatory in these settings. Finally, by challenging traditional concepts about contact investigations and expanding the definition of close contacts to include social contacts and others previously thought to be at lower risk of infection, many more recently infected individuals who are at an increased risk of developing tuberculosis will be identified. This chapter provides a brief background on the rationale for the treatment of latent infection and addresses these priority areas for the prevention of tuberculosis.

TREATMENT OF LATENT TUBERCULOSIS INFECTION

Shortly after the discovery of isoniazid in 1952, the potential of this highly bactericidal drug to prevent tuberculosis was explored. A series of trials summarized in a review by Ferebee (1970) showed that the effectiveness of isoniazid for the prevention of tuberculosis ranged from 92 percent in an outbreak among Dutch sailors, in which adherence to the regimen was strictly enforced (Veening, 1968), to 26 percent in a Tunisian community-based study in which the rate of adherence to the isoniazid regimen was estimated to be only 25 percent or less. A study of 3-, 6-, and 12-month regimens showed that a 12-month regimen was the superior regimen (International Union Against Tuberculosis, 1982) and Comstock (1999) recently presented an analysis that showed that a regimen of at least 9 months likely gives maximum protection.

Isoniazid can cause hypersensitivity reactions, paresthesia, and other adverse effects, but concerns about isoniazid hepatotoxicity have limited the use of isoniazid in the past for the treatment of latent infection. However, this controversy concerns the provision of isoniazid to individuals at relatively low risk of tuberculosis. In contrast, the use of isoniazid has never been challenged for individuals at high risk of tuberculosis, including recent tuberculin skin test converters, contacts of infectious patients, immigrants from countries with high rates of tuberculosis, and individuals with certain medical conditions, especially human immunodeficiency virus (HIV) infection. A recent 7-year study of patients receiving isoniazid for treatment of latent infection showed a rate of clinical hepatitis of only 0.1 percent (11 cases among 11,141 patients), with no deaths and only one hospitalization in a program with patient monitoring, the administration of only limited amounts of medication at each visit, and good education on the symptoms of adverse effects (Nolan et al., 1999).

In addition to isoniazid, rifampin-based regimens have recently been recommended as treatment for latent infection with *M. tuberculosis* (American Thoracic Society, 2000). The current recommended regimens for treatment of latent infection include isoniazid for 9 months (with an option for 6 months), rifampin and pyrazinamide for 2 months, and rifampin alone for 4 months (ATS/CDC statement). Although the rifampin-pyrazinamide regimen has the advantage of being much shorter, the experience with this regimen is relatively limited, and one pilot study that evaluated this regimen showed that it has a very high rate of toxicity. In particular, this regimen has not been evaluated with immigrant populations, and programs that use the regimen are encouraged to maintain surveillance for adverse reactions to this regimen.

CURRENT SCREENING FOR IMMIGRANTS TO THE UNITED STATES

As noted in Chapter 1, increasingly large proportion of tuberculosis cases in the United States occur among foreign-born individuals: 7,591 (41.3 percent) cases in 1998. If the number of U.S.-born individuals with tuberculosis continues to decrease at a rate of 9 percent, as it did between 1992 and 1998, and the number of foreign-born individuals with tuberculosis remains the same, the majority of tuberculosis cases will occur among foreign-born individuals from 2002 onward. The CDC Working Group on Tuberculosis Among the Foreign-Born thus concluded that the elimination of tuberculosis in the United States will increasingly depend on the elimination of tuberculosis among foreign-born individuals.

Foreign-born individuals comprise those who arrive in the United States through a number of mechanisms. The majority who come to the

United States legally are in the United States temporarily. These arrivals include tourists, students and their families, and workers and their families. Immigrants include those who intend to reside permanently in the United States, some who have newly arrived from their country of origin, and others who adjust their status to permanent residency while they are already in the United States.

Tuberculosis is one condition for which immigrants are screened before they enter the United States. This screening currently consists of a chest radiograph for all immigrants 15 years of age and older and the examination of three sputum samples for acid-fast bacilli (AFB) for all individuals with chest radiograph findings consistent with tuberculosis. Immigrants younger than 15 years of age who are suspected of having tuberculosis or of having contact with an individual with a known case of tuberculosis are given a tuberculin skin test, and those with any indication of tuberculosis are given a chest radiograph.

Individuals with any sputum tests positive for AFB are classified as infectious and as having a Class A medical condition. This means that either they must complete an approved course of tuberculosis treatment before entering the United States or that they must start therapy and have three consecutive negative sputum tests before coming to the United States. Individuals who do not complete therapy must have a relative arrange for treatment at the intended destination in the United States, with the concurrence of the local or state tuberculosis control program. They are to be given 30 days of medication when they depart for the United States.

Individuals who have abnormal chest radiograph and sputum examinations but who are negative for AFB are classified as having a Class B medical condition: Class B1 if the radiograph indicates active disease but the individual is not infectious due to negative sputum smears or if the individual has extrapulmonary tuberculosis (such individuals are to be started on therapy and given 30 days of medication before coming to the United States); Class B2 if the radiograph indicates tuberculosis that is not clinically active; and Class B3 if the radiograph indicates old or healed tuberculosis. Individuals with Class B1 or B2 tuberculosis are told to report to the public health department at their final destination.

Any Class A or B medical classification is recorded on immigration documents (DQ [Division of Quarantine] form 75.17). If the immigrant enters one of the eight ports (Honolulu, Seattle, San Francisco, Los Angeles, Chicago, Miami, Atlanta, and New York) where U.S. Public Health Service Division of Quarantine staff are assigned, the quarantine officer gives the immigrant a form that reminds the individual of the requirement to report to the local public health department upon arrival at the final destination. The quarantine officer sends DQ form 75.17 to the CDC Division of Quarantine, which then forwards the forms to state and local health departments. If the immigrant arrives in a port without a quarantine officer, the immigration officer is to collect the form (DQ form 75.17), notify the immigrant of the requirement to report to the local public health department upon arrival at the final destination, and then send DQ form 75.17 to the nearest port with a quarantine officer. There has been no evaluation of the rate of referral of immigration forms from ports without a quarantine officer, but it is believed that many of the forms are not collected and that when they are collected they are often held for long periods of time and sent to a port with a quarantine office in batches.

When the immigration forms are collected and sent to health departments, the follow-up rate of screening of immigrants for tuberculosis can be quite high. It has been estimated to exceed 82 percent in most areas of the United States (Binkin et al., 1996), and one tuberculosis control program has documented a follow-up program that achieved a 97.5 percent follow-up rate (Catlos et al., 1998). However, it costs the program $13–$14 immigrant to follow-up each new arrival and to encourage the individual to report for examination, and the program accounts only for those immigrants about whom the health department was notified by the Division of Quarantine.

THE NEED FOR EXPANDED SCREENING

More than a quarter (29.6 percent) of all cases of tuberculosis among foreign-born individuals occur during the first year after their arrival in the United States, and more than half (55.5 percent) occur during their first 5 years in the United States. The risk for developing tuberculosis declines the longer an immigrant from a country with a high risk of infection is in the United States, because they are no longer at a high risk of infection or reinfection. While the risk of developing tuberculosis for a recently arrived immigrant from a country with a high risk of infection is lower than that of a newly infected person, the risk for the typical immigrant from a high-risk country is many times that of the typical U.S. resident. The current screening procedure for immigrants does not and cannot detect or prevent many of the cases of tuberculosis that occur among foreign-born individuals in the United States. Recent immigrants from countries with high rates of tuberculosis have been identified as prime candidates for screening and treatment of latent infection (American Thoracic Society, 2000), but public health efforts to confront the problem have been inadequate (Binkin et al., 1996). The Working Group on Tuberculosis Among the Foreign-Born concluded,

Efforts to provide screening and preventive therapy for the foreign-born are limited. Averting future cases of TB [tuberculosis] requires linking screening programs to prevention services. However, few resources are available to health departments for prevention efforts to foreign-born persons. Also, persons who do not consider themselves ill and who are from countries where TB is reported as a stigma might be reluctant to begin or complete therapy (Centers for Disease Control and Prevention, 1998:7)

In the current system, the burden is on the health departments to encourage individuals to be screened for tuberculosis infection after they arrive in the United States.

Given the significance of tuberculosis among foreign-born individuals and given the contribution that addressing the incidence of tuberculosis among foreign-born individuals would make to the goal of tuberculosis elimination, the committee believes that the federal government should fund a coordinated national effort to screen foreign-born individuals for tuberculosis. Reliance on the efforts and resources of local health departments unfairly burdens those communities within which a disproportionate number of foreign-born individuals reside, fails to reflect the national interest in radically reducing the rate of tuberculosis among immigrants and refugees, and virtually ensures that the level of commitment will be inadequate for the task.

The strategies that must be developed are linked to the impediments to identifying those with latent tuberculosis infection and ensuring their completion of treatment for latent infection, the sheer size of the populations to be screened, the difficulties in gaining access to those who should be screened, and the cultural and linguistic barriers that make voluntary approaches to screening and treatment of limited utility. A significant departure from current methods of screening and treatment of latent tuberculosis infection among foreign-born individuals is dictated by the clear public health benefits that could be attained.

Strategies to Ensure Case Identification and Treatment Completion

A first step would be to expand the current screening of those applying to immigrate and the screening of refugees. Tuberculin skin testing for latent infection should be added to the current panel of tests used to screen for active tuberculosis (chest radiographs and sputum analysis), and a Class B4 (or other designation) should be created for individuals with a normal chest radiograph but a positive tuberculin skin test. Such testing, like other medical examinations, would occur before the immigrant or refugee came to the United States. Tuberculin skin testing already occurs in the United States for those seeking to adjust their status after coming to the United States on temporary visas. Given the small number of tuberculosis infections detected by tuberculin skin test screening among low-risk populations and the recent recommendations of the American Thoracic Society and the CDC that screening for latent infection be targeted to those at risk, there is little justification for screening all applicants for immigration. Targeting of screening to those who come from countries with the greatest tuberculosis burdens (prevalence of infection estimated to be equal to or greater than the global median of 36 percent) would detect the greatest number of infections and would require the testing of approximately 200,000 immigrants per year. Individuals born in countries with the greatest burdens of tuberculosis account for 55 percent of the cases of tuberculosis among the foreign-born individuals each year. In particular, even though Mexico is estimated to have only a 17 percent prevalence of tuberculosis infection, Mexican-born individuals account for nearly one-quarter of the foreign-born individuals with tuberculosis each year and just under 10 percent of the total number of individuals with tuberculosis in the United States. Requiring immigrants from Mexico to be skin tested before immigration would add about 53,000 immigrants to the testing program each year, increasing the total number of immigrants to be skin tested each year to about 250,000. Among each annual cohort of immigrants from countries with the greatest tuberculosis burdens, approximately 2,100 cases of tuberculosis can be expected to occur over the course of a cohort's first 5 years in the United States. Assuming a steady influx of immigrants, this rate of tuberculosis among each cohort translates into 2,100 cases per year among the population of immigrants who arrived in the past 5 years. As noted in Appendix E, data on the rate of tuberculosis among immigrants have a number of limitations, and estimates obtained by using more recent population and immigration estimates from the 2000 census would be valuable.

Identifying and Treating Latent Infection

The methodology for estimating the number of cases that could be expected to occur among foreign-born individuals, the number of cases that could be prevented by treatment of latent infection, and the costs of a program for the treatment of individuals with latent infection are contained in Appendix E. Assuming an overall rate of effectiveness of treatment for latent infection of 75 percent (allowing for nonadherence), at least 1,300 cases of tuberculosis could be prevented per year during the first 5 years that the immigrants are in the United States. (The number of cases prevented in later years, when the immigrants are at a lower risk of developing tuberculosis, was not estimated.) Overall program costs would be about $23 million per year, and the cost per case of tuberculosis prevented would be about $14,559, which is less than the cost of treating a patient with tuberculosis and monitoring the contacts of that patient, which is $16,391. If the results of the tuberculin skin testing before immigration were accepted and the test was not repeated, the program costs would drop to about $12,305 per case of tuberculosis prevented.

Additional savings will be realized if all individuals with a Class B tuberculosis designation were required to report for tuberculosis screening in the United States. As noted above, tuberculosis control programs are very successful in getting immigrants with a Class B tuberculosis designation to report for examination. However, although such screening is cost-effective, it is costly, and screening of foreign-born individuals with Class B tuberculosis would account for about 12 percent of the tuberculin skin testing costs described above. Shifting the burden to report for screening to the arriving immigrant would reduce the need for intensive follow-up, and the cost per case of tuberculosis prevented could be reduced to $12,920 if all immigrants reported without follow-up.

One method of requiring examination for tuberculosis and tuberculosis infection would be to withhold the "green card" for all immigrants with a Class A or Class B tuberculosis designation and to issue this permanent residency document only when these individuals have completed screening by the health department and treatment (if indicated). This approach may shift costs from the public health programs to the Immigration and Naturalization Service (INS), but the immigrants would have a strong incentive to comply. However, the service may not be as costly if modern information technology is applied. At a minimum, the failure of an immigrant with a Class B tuberculosis designation to report to the health department for screening could be made grounds for deportation, as is already the case for immigrants with a Class A designation and a waiver to enter the United States.

Issues and Concerns

The committee carefully considered the issues surrounding tuberculin skin testing and treatment of latent infection for newly arrived immigrants. An extra public session was added to the committee's schedule to allow a roundtable discussion of the ethical, legal, and practical issues of implementing these programs. After these discussions the committee concluded that the difficulties in implementing the program were largely structural but that these could be overcome with a sufficient commitment of resources. Although these costs will be significant, many of the benefits will accrue to the general programs of targeted tuberculin skin testing and the treatment of individuals with latent infection. Significant additional funding will be required for (a) CDC to provide training and monitor the quality of the tuberculin testing programs, (b) CDC and INS to ensure that information on the immigrants is collected accurately and is promptly communicated to the relevant health departments in the United States, and (c) the state and local health departments that will have to provide the final medical examination and that will be responsible for completion of therapy, when treatment is indicated, including start-up costs for training and infrastructure. However, improvements are needed in the current system of testing for and treatment of latent infections, and this new program could pave the way for a broad array of needed changes. Because of the magnitude of the changes required by this recommendation, the committee suggests that this be implemented in a stepwise approach and that pilot programs be developed to evaluate strategies and assess their costs.

The adoption of a mandatory tuberculin skin test screening program may trouble those concerned with the human rights of immigrants and refugees, foreign workers, and students. In a national climate characterized by occasional hostility to immigrants and assumptions about the burdens posed by foreign-born individuals, it is not difficult to understand such concerns. Nevertheless, the committee can see no fundamental reason why the logic of current tuberculosis screening should not be extended to those with latent infection. Although the threat to the public health from latent infection is not as immediate as the threat that stems from active disease, the overall epidemiological burden is significant. It is that potential burden that justifies such screening.

Treatment of Latent Infections

No program of mandatory screening for latent infection could be justified unless it were linked to a program of treatment of latent infection. Recent analyses have made clear that with isoniazid monotherapy, the recommended course of therapy should be isoniazid therapy daily or twice weekly for 9 months (American Thoracic Society, 2000). A two-drug regimen of rifampin and pyrazinamide daily for as little as 2 months has also been shown to be effective at reducing the risk of disease by the same amount as the 9-month isoniazid regimen, but as noted earlier, toxicity may be an issue for the rifampin-pyrazinamide regimen. For both the long-term monotherapy and the short-course, 2-month regimens, strict adherence to the treatment regimen is crucial.

A positive tuberculin skin test should not impede the entrance of immigrants, refugees, workers and students to the United States. Should the treatment of latent infection, however, be voluntary or mandatory? Reluctance to mandate treatment of latent infection is rooted in concerns about the risks associated with such treatment as well as in constitutional and ethical principles. As noted above, early experience with isoniazid treatment raised questions about its hepatotoxicity. However, it has always been clear that the benefits of isoniazid treatment outweigh the risks of toxicity for those at high risk of tuberculosis. Recent experience has made clear that careful clinical monitoring and the exclusion of those at very high risk of hepatotoxicity can radically reduce the risks associated with treatment of latent infection. Nevertheless, the risks are not absent. These lingering risks, however, along with concerns for individual rights, no longer justify the basic claim for relying solely on voluntary treatment programs.

Payment for Treatment and Community Support

Although the committee acknowledges the importance of protecting and respecting the rights of immigrants and refugees, it believes that the vast public health benefit that would follow from universal treatment of those with latent infection, as recommended by the American Thoracic Society, justifies the imposition of therapy. The federal government, in recognition of the fact that such therapy is primarily designed to achieve a public health goal of national importance, should pay for the treatment of immigrants and refugees. Although the payment for treatment should be from public funds, the provision of treatment should be undertaken in a range of settings. Given the cultural and linguistic barriers that confront individuals who have newly arrived in the United States, much might well be attained by engaging the cooperation of community-based organizations that provide services to distinct ethnic immigrant communities. Certainly such organizations will have much to offer local tuberculosis control programs that may be called upon to provide treatment of newly arrived immigrants for latent infections.

Nonpermanent Residents

Screening of immigrants for latent tuberculosis infection and treatment (if necessary) will not affect students, workers, and their families who come to the United States for long-term stays but do not seek permanent residence. In 1996, 280,000 new arrivals from countries with a high incidence of tuberculosis were students, workers, and their families, and an additional 2,000 cases of tuberculosis per year may occur among these individuals during their first 5 years in the United States. The estimated number of these cases is smaller than that for permanent visa applicants because of differences in the incidence of tuberculosis in their countries of origin. This also is likely to be an overestimate of the number of cases as many of these people would not be in the United States for the full 5 years, and the age distribution of those with immigrant visas (which included the very young and the very old) and those with student and work visas is very different. Health screening is not required for students and workers coming to the United States, and starting a screening program would require a more detailed analysis of the tuberculosis risk for this population. However, school- and employment-based screening and treatment programs should be considered for these new arrivals.

Focusing on those who will be coming to the United States in the future will not address the problem of the estimated 7 million foreign-born individuals with tuberculosis infection already in the United States legally. For them, many of whom are already citizens and the vast proportion of whom may not know of their latent infections, and for all others not screened on entry, programs of culturally sensitive and linguistically appropriate aggressive outreach will be necessary. Programs of mandatory screening would be difficult to launch, as would efforts at imposing mandatory treatment. A close interaction with the private sector, neighborhood health centers, and community-based organizations are going to be necessary if these programs are going to be practical and effective. Skin testing and treatment for latent infection are a part of the *Guide to Clinical Preventive Services* (DHHS, 1996) and individuals from high-risk populations, covered by Medicare will commonly be treated in the private sector. Immigrants from high-risk populations, especially immigrants, are likely to obtain care from neighborhood health centers and community-based organizations and an example of a successful collaboration with the health department in Seattle/King County is noted above. It is the process of immigration that provides a unique opportunity for screening and treatment. It is a process that provides a singular opportunity to advance the goal of tuberculosis elimination.

MANDATORY SCREENING AND TREATMENT OF LATENT INFECTION IN PRISONS AND OTHER CONGREGATE SETTINGS

If much could be achieved in terms of the goal of tuberculosis elimination through a program of mandatory screening and treatment of individuals newly arrived in the United States, considerable benefit would also follow from such screening efforts in congregate settings, where the rates of tuberculosis are historically high: homeless shelters and prisons (see the box Tuberculosis in a Custodial Setting). Prison authorities have an affirmative constitutional duty to protect inmates from infectious conditions (Greifinger et al., 1993). That duty extends not only to the provision of care but also to screening. In 1981, a federal appeals court held that the failure to screen new inmates for communicable conditions violated

Immigrant Outreach and Treatment of Latent Infection

Foreign-born individuals are at the highest risk of latent tuberculosis in their first 5 years in the United States. This provides an opportunity for treatment of latent tuberculosis infection prevention of disease. In King County, Washington, for example, approximately two-thirds of cases of tuberculosis occur among foreign-born individuals. With the assistance of the Annie E. Casey Foundation and the Firland Foundation, the Office of Refugee and Immigrant Assistance of the State of Washington, the Seattle/King County Health Department, and the Community Housecalls and International Medicine Clinic at Harborview Medical Center have engaged in a pilot program of immigrant outreach to increase the effectiveness of tuberculosis screening and prevention services among new refugees and immigrants.

A key component of this program has been the employment of bilingual-bicultural community members who are in good standing in their own community and who are trained to address tuberculosis-related public health and infection control questions. The outreach workers are able to address compliance concerns by providing information about tuberculosis and its transmission and treatment and by assisting with the logistics of medicine pick-up and clinic visits. They provide newly arrived immigrants a cultural as well as a linguistic link to the health care system. The outreach workers also provide newly arrived families information about immigration issues, social welfare regulations, the school system, and access to general health care.

Another key feature of the program has been the use of individual interviews and focus groups with community members on a community-by-community basis. During these interviews and group discussions the symptoms of tuberculosis, the social significance of the disease, the implications of therapy, the concerns about chronic illness in that community, and information about taking medication in the absence of illness are discussed in culture-specific terms that could affect tuberculosis control. After characterizing areas of potential misunderstanding and conflict, tuberculosis health education materials are developed to help the outreach workers (and other health care providers) negotiate these problem areas. (Materials are available via the Internet at http://healthlinks.washington.edu/clinical/ethnomed.)

The program has been extremely successful. At the time of the latest evaluation 89 immigrants from Albania, Bosnia, Ethiopia, Russia, Somalia, Ukraine, Vietnam, and other countries had been started on treatment for latent infection. Five individuals moved, 2 stopped medication on their own initiative, 26 are still on medication, and 53 have successfully completed a 6-month course of therapy. That is an 88 percent (53/60) completion rate for those who could have finished therapy and a 96 percent (53/55) completion rate for those who were eligible to complete therapy and who remained in the area. This success far exceeds the 60–70 percent completion rates obtained by routine programs and has been obtained with a population in whom completion of treatment for latent infection is considered to be particularly difficult.

A formal evaluation of the program will be conducted, including an assessment of its costs, but sensitivity to cultural and linguistic issues must be central to its success. Another important aspect of this pilot project has been the demonstration of a successful collaboration between public-sector, academic, and charitable, nongovernmental organizations in its development and implementation. This model of the delivery of treatment for latent infection and of success in the eradication of tuberculosis that is achievable with foreign-born individuals is worthy of attention.

Tuberculosis in a Custodial Setting

Custodial settings such as prisons can provide two important functions to society toward tuberculosis elimination. Careful monitoring of tuberculosis in these settings provides an early warning of what is occurring in the general public. This was so with the occurrence of multidrug-resistant (MDR) tuberculosis, which was first identified in New York State prisons. In addition, it is much easier to treat tuberculosis while those identified as having infection or disease are institutionalized than when they are again free, as most of them will be.

There are several reasons why the risk of tuberculosis is higher in these settings than in the general public. Those who are incarcerated or institutionalized tend to have more risk factors associated with tuberculosis, factors such as lower socioeconomic status, minority status, abuse of alcohol or other substances, and previously inadequate health care. In addition, institutions place these people who are at higher risk in close contact, often in older, poorly ventilated buildings, facilitating transmission of *M. tuberculosis* when cases of disease occur.

The New York State Department of Correctional Services took the situation in 1991 as a challenge and has shown significant progress. Approximately 25 percent of incoming inmates were infected with *M. tuberculosis;* that rate did not change during the subsequent decade. What did change was the development and spread of active disease. Tuberculosis disease incidence was 225 cases per 100,000 population in 1991. In 1998 it was 40. (This rate includes all individuals with tuberculosis in the system, including those transferred in [15/100,000] and those diagnosed while they were in the system [25/100,000]. The latter rate is similar to the 21/100,000 rate for New York City, from which three-quarters of inmates in the New York State prison system come). Although there were 39 MDR cases of tuberculosis in 1991, there was only 1 in 1998. The rate of new infections within the prison system has been decreased from 1.7 percent in 1993 to 0.25 percent in 1998 for staff and from 2.4 percent to 1.2 percent for inmates. Departmental commitment included staff dedicated to dealing with infectious diseases, mandatory education about tuberculosis and other infectious diseases for all staff and inmates, mandatory skin testing of every one in the system (inmates and staff) mandatory evaluation of all individuals with suspect cases, liberal use of respiratory isolation including all individuals awaiting sputum testing results, directly observed therapy with all antituberculosis medications, and mandatory treatment of latent infection. During the decade more than 750,000 skin tests were given.

Since the New York State corrections system releases nearly 30,000 people back into the general population every year, surveillance, treatment of latent infection, and treatment while in the system provide significant benefits to society. Continuous monitoring will continue to detect significant shifts in the general population.

the Eighth Amendment's prohibition against cruel and unusual punishment since it would expose prisoners to a preventable threat to their health (*Lareau* v. *Manson*, 651 F. 2d 96, 109 [2nd Cir 1981]). In its decision the court wrote that the "resulting threat to the well being of inmates is so serious . . . that this practice constitutes 'punishment' in violation of the

Due Process Clause." A decade later, in the midst of growing alarm about the resurgence of tuberculosis and well-publicized concerns about multi-drug-resistant tuberculosis outbreaks in institutional settings, a federal district court in Pennsylvania mandated that state authorities initiate a tuberculosis control program that included mandatory tuberculin skin test screening (*Austin* v. *Pennsylvania Department of Corrections*, WL 277511 [E.D. Pa. 1992]).

It is thus clear that mandatory screening for latent tuberculosis infection would not only be permissible in prisons but could be required as a matter of law. Such a screening program, however, could be justified only if follow-up therapy for latent tuberculosis infection was available. Could such treatment be mandatory, or might the ethical principle of autonomy and the constitutional right to privacy preclude such an approach, permitting only the offer of treatment? The answer has not been clear.

There is no question that prison authorities would have the authority to impose treatment for communicable conditions. However, can they impose prophylactic interventions? In at least one federal court decision, it was held that prison authorities could require inmates to undergo immunization against diphtheria-tetanus (*Zaire* v. *Dalsheim*, 698 F. Supp, 57 [S.D.N.Y., 1988]). Using an exacting standard of review, the court held that an inmate's privacy interest did not preclude compulsory vaccination because there was "a compelling state interest in preventing the spread of deadly disease among a closely quartered population." Nevertheless, writing in 1993, the director of the prison health system in New York State rejected mandatory treatment of latent tuberculosis infection (Greifinger et al., 1993). It would be "virtually impossible" to compel the taking of oral medication. It would be hard to justify quarantining those who required such treatment because latent infection posed no immediate threat to the health of others. Additionally, there were the clinical risks associated with isoniazid therapy. "Since the risk of developing tuberculosis is low among immunocompetent young adults, the risk of coercive treatment of latent infection appears to outweigh the benefit." Just 3 years later, a successor New York state prison system health director adopted a policy of compulsory treatment for latent tuberculosis infection. His analysis came to a distinctly different conclusion about the risks and benefits involved.

He determined that screening for latent infection without mandated treatment of latent infection for those who are infected inadequately protected the health of the community: the prison community and the wider community. This was consistent with the opinion of the federal court (*Jolly* v. *Coughlin*, 76 F3d 468 [2nd Cir 1996]). To overcome the logistical problems of mandatory skin testing and treatment for latent infection, while at the same time protecting the health of the community and the constitutional rights of the inmates, a new status, "tuberculin hold," was established. Those who decline or who are unable to meet the mandatory requirements are restricted to their cells with careful monitoring for clinical or X-ray signs of disease for 1 year. The length of this status was determined on the basis of the greater risk of development of disease in the first year after infection, with the year based on the worst-case scenario that infection occurred at the time of refusal of the mandated testing and treatment of latent infection. (To meet constitutional requirements, inmates on "tuberculin hold" are provided with 1 hour of outdoor recreation time per day.) Confining inmates to their cells limits the potential spread of tuberculosis if disease should develop, but it is less restrictive than respiratory isolation, which is required in the case of inmates with disease.

The current tuberculosis control policy of the New York State Department of Correctional Services has been reviewed by a federal court, where it has been found not to violate inmates' constitutional rights (*Word* v. *Wright*, 98-CV-220 [U.S. District Court for the Western District of New York]).

Given the state of prison health care systems and the potential for abuse of prisoners, any proposal for mandatory treatment must be subject to careful review from constitutional and ethical perspectives. Given the long-term strategy of tuberculosis elimination, the relative safety of carefully monitored treatment of latent infection, the risks to prisoners—both HIV-infected prisoner and other prisoners—of exposure to tuberculosis in overcrowded settings, and policy initiatives that extend the treatment of tuberculosis infection to nonincarcerated populations, the committee concludes that a program of mandatory prophylactic treatment in prisons will serve the interests of both inmate populations and the public health more broadly.

EXPANDING CONTACT INVESTIGATIONS AND IMPROVING OUTBREAK MANAGEMENT

CDC estimates that an average investigation of each case of tuberculosis in the United States results in the identification of approximately nine close contacts. On average, 30 percent of contacts are infected and another 1 percent will have already progressed to active disease. Approximately 5–10 percent of those with latent infection (depending on the length of time since infection) will progress from latent infection to active disease, and half of these cases will occur during the first 2 years after exposure. The prevalence of tuberculosis among close contacts is approximately 700 per 100,000 population (nearly 100-fold higher than that in the general population) (Binkin et al., 1999; Moodie and Riley, 1974). Therefore, the examination of contacts or persons exposed to an individual with tuberculosis is one of the most important methods of case finding for either tuberculosis disease or latent infection.

The transmission of tuberculosis to contacts has been documented in many diverse locations such as institutions (CDC, 1987), doctor's offices (Askew et al., 1997), airplanes (Kenyon et al., 1996), crack houses (CDC, 1991), HIV respite facilities (Daley et al., 1992), drug rehabilitation centers (CDC, 1980), navy ships (DiStasio and Trump, 1990), and renal transplant units (Jereb et al., 1993). The utility and importance of contact investigations in these settings and for high-risk groups such as foreign-born individuals (Wells et al., 1997) and children under 15 years of age (Casanova et al., 1991; Fernandez et al., 1994; Goldman et al., 1994; Mehta and Bentley, 1992; Rubilar et al., 1995; Topley et al., 1996) and follow-up of patients with multidrug-resistant tuberculosis cases (CDC, 1987; Snider et al., 1985) have also been demonstrated. In addition, it has been shown that the rate of adherence to treatment for latent tuberculosis infection may be highest among contacts (Menzies et al., 1993).

In the United States, health departments currently perform 90 percent of the contact tracing investigations (Binkin et al., 1999). These investigations, as noted above, are the second highest priority (after the early identification and treatment of individuals with active tuberculosis) for tuberculosis control programs. As cases of tuberculosis have retreated into defined pockets of the population (e.g., geographic and risk behavior groups), it has become necessary to modify traditional contact tracing epidemiology to address the specific needs of the individuals in these groups. The contact tracing investigation may now include other types of domiciles such as homeless shelters, correctional facilities, nursing homes, and HIV hospices.

As all cases of tuberculosis began by contact with an individual with tuberculosis, use of a strategy of the early identification and evaluation of contacts and completion of treatment for latent tuberculosis infection would clearly move the country toward tuberculosis elimination. Unfortunately, even in a country as rich with resources as the United States, contact investigations are often less than successful. The literature offers numerous examples of both highly productive and less than adequate contact investigations (Allos et al., 1996; Barnes et al., 1991; Hedemark, 1996; Holcombe, 1996; Hussain et al., 1992; Peerbooms et al., 1995; Sasaki et al., 1995). In addition, several recent outbreaks of tuberculosis have highlighted the need for enhanced efforts to prevent transmission (Allos et al., 1996; Bock et al., 1998; Kenyon et al., 1997; Mangura et al., 1998; Nivin et al., 1998; Valway et al., 1998; Washko et al., 1998).

The goals of a contact investigation are to identify exposed individuals who may have infection or disease and ensure that they are screened and monitored as appropriate, identify the source of tuberculosis disease transmission (this is particularly relevant for children with active tuberculosis when recent transmission is likely), and identify a tuberculosis outbreak when more newly infected persons or more tuberculosis cases are discovered during the investigation than were anticipated on the basis of previous epidemiological data. In this situation, contact tracing may then lead to expanded outbreak investigation activities.

The problems associated with contact investigations that must be addressed to achieve improvements in the effectiveness of these investigations are grouped into eight specific areas, which are identified and described in the following sections.

Public Health Infrastructure

As stated in an article in *Pennsylvania Medicine,*

> Contact investigation is very likely the least appreciated of the activities of any tuberculosis program or clinic. It requires highly educated tuberculosis staff who have experience to deal with the different situations that occur as a result of a case of pulmonary tuberculosis coming to detection. . . . In the year described, thousands of hours of staff time were required to perform the contact work. It is unrealistic to conceive that such work could be performed by any other group than a dedicated and knowledgeable tuberculosis staff, without losing quality of performance and without incurring much greater cost and illness. (Rubin and Lynch, 1996)

A declining public health infrastructure is one problem that may affect either the ability of a tuberculosis control program to respond in a timely manner or the capacity to achieve a response (Barnes et al., 1991; Marks et al., 1999). Anticipated decreases in funding and the attendant downsizing, staff turnover, and inexperience will affect a tuberculosis control program's ability to respond effectively and to prioritize its activities. In addition, as the numbers of cases of tuberculosis decline, it is a reasonable expectation that the responsibilities of public health staff may be shifted elsewhere. When tuberculosis control resources are scarce (as in low-incidence areas), decisions about who will respond (a public health nurse, epidemiologist, or outreach staff) and who will supervise the effort must be made. Inadequate resources may lead to the assignment of untrained staff to many contact investigation tasks. As is demonstrated in the case study in the box Tale of Two Counties, these same limitations can profoundly affect an area's ability to stop the transmission of tuberculosis in an outbreak situation.

Tale of Two Counties

In 1994, an outbreak of tuberculosis occurred in two rural counties in two adjacent states that had each previously reported less than one case of tuberculosis per year. The extent of contact investigation follow-up varied considerably between both counties, as did the results (Onorato, 1999).

Summary of outcomes:

	County A	County B
Percentage of contacts screened	65	98
Percentage who completed isoniazid treatment	54	74
Number of secondary cases	10	0

The differences between the two counties included the fact that County B used creative approaches, had culturally sensitive staff, used on-site directly observed therapy or directly observed preventive therapy, maintained better confidentiality, and provided education for local health care providers. In addition, the links between the health department and the community were stronger in County B.

This experience demonstrated the need for a long-term approach and long-term support in low-incidence areas. Contact investigation and outbreak management can be extremely complex, and increasing numbers of public health jurisdictions will be unprepared as tuberculosis becomes rarer.

Contact Investigation Factors

Attitudinal beliefs and social or cultural differences between the health department staff and the patient or the patient's contacts can affect the staff's ability to conduct an effective investigation. The overriding influences of socioeconomic factors (e.g., homelessness, intravenous drug use, and cultural and linguistic barriers) require new strategies. Culturally sensitive and diverse staff are increasingly needed at all levels of investigation and monitoring. Similarly, staff who are skilled in identifying risk factors for HIV infection during the interview process are needed so that a contact's risk of developing tuberculosis can be properly assessed.

It is also important to clearly determine the responsibilities of the field investigator. Jurisdictions vary in the person assigned to carry out field investigation tasks. Some require assessment by a nurse, whereas others allow outreach staff to administer skin tests and collect sputum specimens from symptomatic patients. Nursing practice issues have been raised, as have liability concerns. On the other hand, resource allocation may be scarce, and the ability to conduct a skin test onsite has distinct advantages.

The failure to recognize an outbreak and to expand an investigation when one is needed can create serious problems (Barnes et al., 1991). Inadequate contact investigations can result in continued transmission of tuberculosis. Missed epidemiological links can have profound consequences as evidenced in a recent outbreak among participants in a floating card game in the rural south (Bock, 1998). (See the box Tuberculosis Outbreak.)

Difficulties can also arise that relate to the size of the setting in which the contact investigation must be conducted (e.g., in homeless shelters, multiple work sites, or airplanes and trains). Public health officials face many challenges in contact investigations that require massive screenings. These include providing sufficient follow-up to personalize the po-

---

Tuberculosis Outbreak in a Floating Card Game in the Rural South: Is the Deck Marked Against Tuberculosis Control?

When nine tuberculosis cases occurred in a rural southern county in an 18-month period (more than had occurred in the previous 10 years combined, with the result being an annual tuberculosis case rate of 86 per 100,000 people), investigators knew they were stumped. An investigation was conducted 19 months after the index patient's case was diagnosed and his acknowledged contacts were evaluated and treated for tuberculosis infection. The investigation revealed that he should also have identified at his initial interview about contacts his two card-playing associates, an extramarital liaison, and another social contact. All four of these individuals presented with tuberculosis disease 7 to 18.5 months later; one of the individuals had HIV coinfection and died. Secondary transmission with additional cases of tuberculosis also occurred. DNA fingerprinting of the available isolates confirmed that the index patient had transmitted the disease to the additional four contacts. Treatment of latent infection could have prevented the progression of their infections to active disease.

State tuberculosis control consultants assisted regional and county staff with evaluating and controlling the outbreak. Three reasons for the inadequate evaluation of case contacts appeared likely. First, local public health workers with limited previous tuberculosis control experience failed to recognize the extent of the exposure and to extend the investigation when a high proportion of contacts were found to be infected. Second, the index patients failed to disclose illegal and illicit social contacts. Third, ethnic minorities were reluctant to participate in a contact investigation conducted by individuals from outside their community.

The outbreak demonstrates the current challenges for tuberculosis control programs in the United States. As the rates of tuberculosis decline, programs will be challenged to maintain expertise among staff who manage few cases. Skilled interviewers are needed to overcome the challenges of ensuring confidentiality when illegal and illicit social connections, such as gambling and drug-using partners, are involved. Another challenge will be to overcome barriers to minority ethnic communities' participation in the health care system.

tential risk and the need for followthrough with public health recommendations and ensuring that skin tests are consistently performed by trained and experienced personnel, particularly when skin test administration and reading of results must be delegated to numerous local health departments and private health care providers. In some settings such as schools, institutions, or work sites, the desire on the part of the employees or administration to overtest individuals to ameliorate the hysteria often associated with knowledge of a case of tuberculosis may influence the direction of the investigation. In addition, pressure exerted by various organizations or groups to protect their members through case isolation or universal testing may be exerted.

Skin testing problems because of false-positive results due to *Mycobacterium bovis* BCG continue to pose obstacles to the contact investigation process. Many foreign-born children were vaccinated with BCG at birth, increasing the possibility of a false-positive test. Also, contacts with a history of BCG vaccination often fail to believe that they are at risk and therefore may not comply with recommendations for testing and treatment. In addition, false-negative tests are possible due to malnourishment, treatment with immunosuppressive drugs, and concomitant disease, such as a childhood infection or HIV infection. The need for the contact to be seen 48–72 hours after testing to have the skin test read can also be problematic for both the contact and the investigator. The need for repeat testing for those contacts who were initially skin test negative 10–12 weeks postexposure (the "window period") adds additional barriers to the completion of the medical evaluation. Location of contacts 3 months later can be difficult, and often, contacts do not see the need for retesting. For health departments that are already stretched for resources, retesting may assume less of a priority.

Finally, the failure to ensure completion of treatment for latent infection will result in a failed contact investigation process, no matter how successful the previous steps were. Data on the completion of treatment for latent infection vary, but data from a recent CDC study suggest that in the states and big cities that it surveyed, the completion-of-therapy rate was 57 percent, but only 44 percent of those who were eligible for therapy completed it. For one-third of those who started therapy, completion-of-therapy status was noted as either "refused/uncooperative" or "unknown." The impact of improving completion of treatment for latent infection can be seen by considering that there were roughly 14,000 people with pulmonary tuberculosis, and at least half of these people would have been smear positive and therefore highly infectious. If each of these cases had 3 infected contacts, there would be 21,000 infected contacts; without any treatment, a conservative estimate would be that 7 percent (the standard estimate of a 10 percent risk minus 3 percent of individuals who may have already developed disease by the time of the investigation) or 1,470 of these people would develop tuberculosis disease. Assuming a 90 percent efficacy of therapy among those who complete treatment, 582 cases of tuberculosis would be prevented if 44 percent of these people completed therapy, while 1,190 cases would be prevented if 90 percent of them completed therapy.

Public Health Resources

Jurisdictions with a high or medium prevalence of tuberculosis would likely find it most efficient to place the responsibility for contact investigations within their health departments. The suggested activities to be maintained by these programs are summarized in Table 4-1.

Jurisdictions with a low prevalence of tuberculosis may not be able to justify use of the public health resources required to maintain all of the suggested activities of a contact investigation listed in Table 4-1, and a secondary support system should be developed. One option would be the establishment of regional response teams. It may be difficult for state tuberculosis program staff to provide on-site expertise to other states, but models of regional and state collaborations for the provision of tuberculosis services currently exist, including long-term hospitalization, education, consultation, and laboratory support. Another approach to regional or state collaboration would be the establishment of a federal "swat" team that would provide an immediate response to an outbreak. Such a federal swat team might overcome some of the problems of the provision of services by staff from one state in another state. Disease investigators from other programs, other appropriately trained staff with alternative duties, or staff with multiple duties could perform the investigations if proper guidance were available. Supervision and evaluation could be provided by properly trained and experienced public health nurses or other designated clinical staff. Regional centers of expertise could be used for consultation and technical assistance.

In states where primary public health responsibility is in counties or similar jurisdictions, vertical responsibility systems could be established. State tuberculosis control programs would be responsible for planning for incremental increases in skills, with local public health staff being responsible for the initiation of case management. Working within a network of more experienced supervisors and consultants, local public health workers could be directed by regional supervisors, who would report to state-level specialists in medicine, nursing, epidemiology, and behavioral and social aspects of tuberculosis case management.

Whether it is a jurisdiction with a high prevalence or a low prevalence of tuberculosis, these responsibilities will require adequate funding (state

TABLE 4-1 Suggested Activities of a Contact Investigation Program

- Administrative direction, support, and commitment
- Establishment of a priority system for identified contacts (CDHS/CTCA, 1998)
- Establishment of a computerized contact registry (Brook et al., 1999)
- Use of confidentiality requirements and training
- Use of a standardized assessment and other procedural tools (CDHS/CTCA, 1998; Kawamura and Green Rush, 1999; Lohuis et al., 1999)
- Assurance of setting-based contact follow-up in the field
- Use of staff education and training
- Use of quality assurance (a comprehensive evaluation system must be in existence for use throughout the process)
- Consideration of legal orders that require the contact to comply with screening and examination recommendations
- Use of staff who understand the social dynamics of the community (ethnography and social networks analysis) and the racial or ethnic barriers to participation
- Mandatory assignment of outreach workers to high-risk contacts and mandatory follow-up home visits
- Use of directly observed preventive therapy for select high-risk contacts such as contacts of a patient with multidrug-resistant tuberculosis
- On-site directly observed preventive therapy for infected contacts
- Use of skilled, culturally and linguistically appropriate interviewers
- Use of restriction fragment length polymorphism analysis (DNA fingerprinting) as a routine adjunct to outbreak investigations
- Inclusion and discussion of contact information and follow-up during routine case conferences
- Use of expanded contact investigation teams and models when needed (Kellogg et al., 1987)
- Availability of rapid smear tests for diagnosis to avoid the unnecessary expense and anxiety related to initiating unwarranted contact investigations
- Connections to and ongoing communication with all reporting sites to encourage reporting of cases and suspected cases in a timely fashion
- Connections to and ongoing communication with community-based organizations, neighborhood health centers, and other medical care providers to ensure that high-risk populations have access to appropriate and adequate contact care

and federal). The commitment to support a comprehensive program to ensure that contacts are identified, provided access to adequate and appropriate care, and monitored until the completion of therapy is a key in the advance toward the elimination of tuberculosis.

Private Providers

Several problems related to management of contact follow-up by private providers that evaluate and treat patients with tuberculosis and their contacts arise. One such problem is the delay in reporting of the case to the health department once it is diagnosed (from a variety of private-sector settings, e.g., hospitals, correctional facilities, and health centers), which may allow continued transmission. Often, private providers fail to recommend treatment for latent tuberculosis infection for contacts at high risk. In the study by Marks et al. (1999), only 50 percent of those close contacts who were at high risk for disease were placed on therapy. Problems related to ensuring public health follow-up activities for patients and contacts monitored in managed care settings are also encountered with private providers.

Although private providers are expected to report cases or suspected cases, the health departments have responsibility for ensuring that they are reported in a timely fashion. Strategies such as the use of 24-hour reporting lines, reporting fact sheets, the use of easy-to-remember or identify reporting telephone numbers, and educational efforts about reporting responsibilities and the role of the health department targeted to physicians in all settings conducted on a routine basis should promote reporting of cases or suspected cases of tuberculosis. Evaluation activities related to reporting, such as validation studies, accuracy of information, review of cases by reporting status, and time to notification could be a routine health department activity for the identification of physicians and institutions that do not report cases of tuberculosis or tuberculosis infection in a timely manner and that should accordingly be contacted.

Health departments can work collaboratively with providers in the private sector to ensure that contacts are placed on treatment and complete their treatment for latent tuberculosis infection. If a contact is identified through the health department tracking system as one who is being monitored by a private-sector provider, educational messages need to be delivered to the providers about the risk for the patient (on the basis of the transmission assessment) and the importance of the patient beginning and completing treatment for latent tuberculosis infection. Health departments should also be tracking contacts seen in the private sector for completion of treatment status and should provide assistance as needed, including directly observed therapy for treatment of latent infection.

As tuberculosis retreats into defined populations in limited geographical areas, physicians will see a tuberculosis case less often in their daily practices, and will be less likely to consider the diagnosis in their initial workup. The CDC revised edition of the Tuberculosis Core Curriculum has a small section on contact investigations and will be a useful reference when it is published. However, additional resources are needed in a format that is accessible to all physicians. As described in the discussion of education and training in Chapter 3, medical school curricula should contain basic information on the diagnosis of tuberculosis, but in some areas, medical expertise in tuberculosis will need to be maintained at a different level through state health departments, hot lines, centers of excellence, and so on.

Lack of Consistent National Policies for Contact Investigations

The only document that suggests a national strategy for contact investigation is the American Thoracic Society-American Lung Association Control Statement written in 1992 (ATS/ALA, 1992). This is outdated in that it does not address the situations, described earlier in the report, that challenge conventional wisdom about tuberculosis transmission. These include transmission in a social situation (the floating card game) and the higher than expected proportion of cases in which transmission occurred from smear-negative individuals, as discussed in Chapter 2. As a result, various tuberculosis control programs use different methods for different aspects of contact investigations.

For example, once a case or a suspected case of tuberculosis is reported, decisions must be made about those cases that require contact tracing. This is often problematic, as in some areas of the country contact investigations are restricted to contacts of smear-positive individuals with pulmonary or laryngeal tuberculosis, whereas in other jurisdictions a broader definition may apply. In addition, as children are rarely infectious, in some areas a contact investigation may be replaced by a source case investigation to identify the person who transmitted disease to the child. Even with new national guidelines about the reporting of contacts (which emphasize smear status), there is still controversy about using smear status as a marker of potential transmission (Barnes, 1998; Behr et al., 1999; Corless et al., 1999; Iseman, 1997; Liippo et al., 1993; Menzies, 1997a,b; Rodriguez et al., 1996). Routine screening of all contacts of patients smear positive for AFB as part of the contact investigation process may be all inclusive but may also waste considerable resources on patients who do not have tuberculosis as their final diagnosis (environmental mycobacteria are also AFB) (Corless et al., 1999). To complicate matters further, transmission from smear-negative patients has also been noted (Behr et al., 1999).

It is also often difficult to define the period of infectiousness. When the contact is unable to remember reliably when his or her symptoms began, some jurisdictions elect to define the period of infectiousness as beginning at least 3 months before treatment started. For other jurisdictions it may be from the time of diagnosis. As there are no guidelines in this regard, there is no consistency in programmatic approach. Other problems include the lack of consistent, standardized definitions for all aspects of the contact investigation process, including definitions of "contact," "close contact," "other-than-close contact," and so on. Documentation problems are common throughout the investigation process (Barnes et al., 1991), and as no standardized methodology for data upkeep, analysis, or evaluation exists or is required, programs approach these tasks differently. Additionally, no national, consensus guidelines for tuberculosis outbreak investigations exist such as response plans or procedures. Tuberculosis programs were required to have an "outbreak response plan" as part of their Year 2000 Cooperative Agreement grant applications for funding from the CDC, but no guidance was given on a standardized approach.

The newly established CDC Contact Working Group could serve as a vehicle to facilitate the development of much needed standardized recommendations and implementation strategies, such as definitions, common elements, and formats for data collection (including factors that place an individual at high risk for tuberculosis and at high risk of a lack of adherence to treatment), methods for assessment of all contacts (tuberculosis skin test positive or negative) for factors that place them at high risk for tuberculosis and prioritization for follow-up on the basis of these factors, methods for ensuring counseling for the prevention of HIV infection and testing for all individuals at risk for HIV infection, methods for determination of the date of last exposure, and evaluation standards. Collaboration with the National Tuberculosis Controllers Association could assist with this process. In addition, current state or big city contact investigation guidelines (where they exist) and other related materials (algorithms, fact sheets, etc.) can be reviewed as potential models or examples.

As part of its global efforts, CDC could work with the International Union Against Tuberculosis and Lung Diseases Nursing Section's International Working Group on Contact Investigations. This group has developed a list of international referrals to be used to monitor contacts who leave the state or country.

Lack of Knowledge About Need for and Importance of Contact Investigations

Contact investigation education has three components: provider education (including public health), patient and contact education, and the patient-provider relationship.

Provider Education

A major difficulty for providers is priority setting. Those who lack training and experience often do not understand the need for a systematic approach to the investigation. Providers may also lack knowledge as to who is at risk of progression to disease, and resources may be spent on delivering services to individuals who are not at demonstrated risk. The lack of a standardized approach to tuberculin skin testing and reading of the results may also result in misinterpretations that may confound the process. Finally, there are failures to recognize an outbreak and to expand an investigation when needed (Barnes et al., 1991).

Patient and Contact Education

A delay in diagnosis may result when a patient with tuberculosis fails to seek treatment. Asch and colleagues (1998) have reported that 30 percent of symptomatic patients with tuberculosis did not obtain medical attention for more than 30 days after the onset of symptoms. This delay adds to the potential for transmission to contacts. The reasons for this delay may include patient or contact mistrust of the government or health care system or related immigration issues. Cultural beliefs that cause fear of stigmatization because of tuberculosis, tuberculosis and HIV coinfection, or other factors may also interfere with the contact investigation process. Patients may be reluctant to divulge contact information if they are worried about the perceptions of others. The lifestyles of many tuberculosis patients result in competing priorities. Drug use or the need for food and shelter for homeless people may take priority over medical care. Although some patients readily provide the names of their contacts, misunderstandings about how tuberculosis is transmitted may lead to misunderstandings of what a true contact is and the patient may inadvertently miss some critical information (Shrestha-Kuwahara et al., 1999). Patients are also often reluctant to identify risk factors for HIV infection. Finally, among foreign-born individuals, there are misconceptions about the receipt and presumed protectiveness of the BCG vaccine. Many of these factors result in the failure of contacts to respond to the screening efforts (Brassard and Lamarre, 1999; Hussain et al., 1992). For example, in a church choir outbreak (Mangura et al., 1998), few persons (less than one-third) who were exposed participated in the initial skin testing and one-third of those who did participate did not return for readings of the skin test results. Similar findings have been found in other settings, such as a pediatric outpatient clinic, where, despite extensive resource dedication, only 43 percent of exposed children completed screening (Moore et al., 1998).

Patient-Provider Relationship

The patient-provider relationship is often complicated by different attitudinal beliefs and social or cultural differences. Either the interviewer, the interviewee, or both may be uncomfortable with the HIV risk assessment questions. Also, as mentioned previously, the patient's perceptions of contact may be different from the provider's epidemiological perceptions of contact with tuberculosis (Booysen et al., 1999).

To overcome all of these obstacles, providers need skills in patient assessment, interviewing, counseling, communication, skin testing, and reading and evaluation. Models exist for some of these areas, such as training courses in contact investigation and interviewing skills offered through CDC-funded Model Tuberculosis Centers. The New Jersey Model Tuberculosis Center, for example, offers improved contact investigation interviewing techniques through innovative skills-based training. If offered on a regional basis (with adequate supportive funding), this type of training would allow more participation and interaction by providers with patients. These courses should also promote the development of skills in basic environmental assessment techniques for use in field investigations. CDC, in conjunction with the Model Tuberculosis Centers, recently offered via the Internet a self-study module on contact investigation that was reportedly quite successful. The CDC also plans to release this material on videotape and as an interactive computer-based course.

Patient and provider educational materials are needed to facilitate the contact investigation process. Educational materials for patients need to be culturally and linguistically appropriate, as well as at the correct level of literacy for the targeted population, and they need to be evaluated to assess their effectiveness. Committee members were not aware of efforts by either CDC or the Model Tuberculosis Centers to develop these materials and encourage their development, along with the other patient educational materials discussed in Chapter 3. Before the development of the educational materials, appropriate theories and models of behavioral change need to be evaluated and used as appropriate to deliver effective, targeted messages, materials, and programs for health care providers and patients.

The patient-provider relationship would be enhanced through cultural awareness training for providers. Some tuberculosis programs have already established such training programs, and these programs or models from other disease control programs should be available to all providers. The patient-provider relationship will also be enhanced by training in skills in counseling for the prevention of HIV infection and testing for HIV infection, which should be widely available to all providers.

Data

The lack of knowledge as to what types of data are needed can significantly affect the quality and performance of the contact investigation. This problem was noted in a study conducted in several state and big city tuberculosis control programs (Marks et al., 1999). Their results indicate that there were great variations as to who was collecting data from the sites surveyed, as well as what information was being obtained. The study noted that less information was recorded for individuals who were tuberculin skin test negative or who did not begin treatment for latent infection, no contacts were noted for many patients with tuberculosis, no notation that identified persons at high risk for disease (especially HIV) was found, and risk factors for nonadherence to treatment were rarely recorded. In a presentation to the committee it was noted that 2 of 11 programs surveyed did not record the date of last exposure to establish time frames for investigation, and no record of follow-up skin tests was noted for 43 percent those who were initially negative (Onorato, 1999).

The lack of general prevalence data on which to base a decision to expand (or not expand) an investigation is also problematic. Although the current expansion of the National Health and Nutritional Examination Survey (NHANES) to include tuberculosis will collect some general prevalence data, given the type of sampling used for that survey, it is questionable whether the results from that survey can be extrapolated for use in contact investigations.

Regarding data accessibility, studies have shown that the inability to obtain information can profoundly affect the results of the investigation (Hussain et al., 1992; Nivin et al., 1998). For example, in a tuberculosis outbreak in a hospital nursery (Nivin et al., 1998) contact investigation difficulties included the fact that inadequate data on tuberculin skin testing of hospital employees were available and many records could not be located at all.

The CDC Working Group on Contact Investigations or a similar group should develop guidelines for data collection: what types of data are needed, where data should be maintained, how many data should be collected, and so on. Guidelines should outline and specify the types of data required for all aspects of the contact investigation process, follow-up, analysis, and evaluation.

There is also a need for community-specific tuberculosis prevalence data, if that is to be the measure used for comparison in the expansion of investigations. If this is not feasible, then alternative means of decision making need to be developed and disseminated. Health departments should work with health care providers to ensure that contact testing data are accessible when they are needed. Laws that allow public health agency access to data for investigations of infectious diseases should be enforced, and provider collaboration with public health agencies should be enhanced.

Framework

The current contact investigation process does not appear to adequately incorporate host susceptibility into the priority-setting process. For example, contacts who are infected with HIV may belong in the first group of contacts evaluated, regardless of the extent of contact. Another factor associated with the determination of host susceptibility relates to the adequacy of HIV risk assessment techniques used during the contact investigation process (particularly for those who are skin test negative) (Barnes et al., 1991; Barnes et al., 1996). If these techniques are not adequate, persons at the highest risk of disease may be missed.

Recent data also suggest that the concentric circle method (i.e., examining groups at lower risk of exposure only if the higher risk group had a high rate of infection) may not completely address contact investigation needs (Bock et al., 1998; Cegielski et al., 1997; Fitzpatrick et al., 1999; Mangura et al., 1998; Rothenberg, 1996). Some of these investigators have suggested that this traditional approach be modified or changed to reflect the influence of social networking. Two recent reports highlight this need. In an investigation of a church choir, all cases of tuberculosis were reported separately by each township in quite diverse communities (Mangura et al., 1998). Traditional contact investigation methods had identified no workplace or family contacts. In the investigation of participants in a floating card game described earlier in this chapter, the failure to identify the existence of numerous social networks propagated the outbreak (Bock et al., 1998). These examples demonstrate the importance of congregate activities outside of work and the importance of assumed socially defined high-risk groups.

The role of DNA fingerprinting in contact investigations needs to be further defined. Three recent reports suggest the importance of molecular epidemiology in understanding the application of the current contact investigation framework. In the first of these, the conventional means of contact investigation failed to identify epidemiological links, in which typing by restriction fragment length polymorphism (RFLP) analysis led to the detection of a community outbreak among HIV-infected persons (Tabet et al., 1994). The common place of transmission was a local bar. A second example was an investigation in Los Angeles in which RFLP analysis showed that the locations at which the homeless population congregate were important sites of tuberculosis transmission for both homeless and nonhomeless people (Barnes et al., 1997). Finally, a study in Baltimore by Bishai and colleagues (1998) suggests that measures to reduce tuberculosis transmission should be location specific instead of based on the concentric circle method. RFLP analysis in the context of contact investigations also raises the issue of reopening such investigations on the basis of new results by RFLP analysis. The costs and benefits must still be assessed to evaluate this strategy.

If research demonstrates that new frameworks for contact investigations such as social networking or location-based screening are effective, health department staff and other providers will require training in their applicability and use. Education on tuberculosis and contact tracing strategies will need to be adapted to the characteristics of distinct population groups. Expansion of screening programs might be applicable for groups at increased risk of transmission, particularly if it seems that traditional contact investigations are not feasible.

Safety and Confidentiality

Safety and confidentiality issues reflect the changing world of tuberculosis and the associated program implications for investigators. Safety for the investigator is an issue, given the high-crime-rate areas where contact investigations are frequently conducted. Decisions need to be made about security, and plans to ensure safety should be developed as needed (Bock et al., 1998). In addition, confidentiality can be difficult to maintain in some settings, particularly during workplace- and institution-based outbreaks.

Research

The lack of a scientific basis for some aspects of the contact investigation process affects the potential effectiveness and efficiency of the investigation and restricts the investigator's ability to stop further transmission of disease. This is particularly true in the determination of transmission factors. As noted earlier, it is still not possible to define precisely the limits of the contact investigation. Although mathematical models for analysis of potential transmission of tuberculosis are available, the factors that affect both the transmission and the acquisition of disease are variable and difficult to calculate (Nardell et al., 1991). For example, there are continued difficulties in defining the extent of "infectiousness."

Although the transmission risk assessment provides some direction, it lacks scientific validation, and some of the variables are open to question (e.g., the relationship between transmission and smear status [as noted earlier], patients with "normal" chest X rays, and the clinical presentation in children) (Barnes, 1998; Behr et al., 1999; Corless et al., 1999; Iseman, 1997; Kenyon et al., 1997; Menzies, 1997a; Pena et al., 1999). Differences in the virulence of the infecting organism also affect transmission. The ability to define such virulence would help the investigator to better prioritize contact efforts by being able to focus on those who are defined as potential "superspreaders" (Valway et al., 1998; van Soolingen et al., 1996; Zhang et al., 1992). The reverse is also true for children, who are not usually considered infectious. A better understanding of transmission factors as they relate to children would assist the investigator in decision making in such difficult settings as schools or day-care centers. A better definition of the protection afforded by the BCG vaccine and its relevance to exposure would also help define those at risk of transmission (Menzies, 1996). There are also continued difficulties in defining environmental factors such as direction of airflow, volume of ventilation, the presence of ultraviolet light, crowding, and volume of air space. Finally, the recent recommendations of ACET suggest that operational research is needed to (a) ensure prompt and complete identification of contacts, (b) increase the numbers of appropriate contacts who are identified, (c) increase the proportion of infected contacts who are placed on treatment for latent infection, and (d) and increase the proportion who complete therapy (CDC, 1999).

Conclusion

If tuberculosis elimination efforts are to be successful, prevention activities must be targeted to the groups at highest risk for progression from tuberculosis infection to disease. Contacts of patients with infectious cases of tuberculosis are such a high-risk group, and the tracing of contacts should be priorities for tuberculosis control programs. Although the focus of contact tracing is prevention, other potential benefits of the investigation may include the identification of additional cases of tuberculosis and the opportunity for education about tuberculosis disease, the risk of transmission, the tuberculosis-HIV connection, and so on. As every case of tuberculosis began as a contact, the ability to rapidly identify tuberculosis cases and to effectively conduct the subsequent contact tracing is one of the cornerstones of tuberculosis control efforts by public health agencies. Without this capacity, transmission of tuberculosis will persist, the decline in the numbers of cases of tuberculosis will stop, and tuberculosis elimination will be impossible to achieve.

REFERENCES

Allos BM, Gensheimer KF, Bloch AB, Parrotte D, Horan JM, Lewis V, and Schaffner W. 1996. Management of an outbreak of tuberculosis in a small community. *Ann Intern Med* 125:114–117.

American Thoracic Society/American Lung Association. 1992. Control of tuberculosis in the United States. *Am Rev Respir Dis* 146:1623–1633.

American Thoracic Society and Centers for Disease Control and Prevention. 2000. Targeted tuberculosis testing and treatment of latent infection. *Am J Respir Crit Care Med* 161:5221–5247.

Asch S, Leake B, Anderson R, and Gelberg L. 1998 Why do symptomatic patients delay obtaining care for tuberculosis? *Am J Respir Crit Care Med* 157:1244–1248

Askew GL, Finelli L, Hutton M, et al. 1997. *Mycobacterium tuberculosis* transmission from a pediatrician to patients. *Pediatrics* 100:19–23.

Barnes PF. 1998. Reducing the ongoing transmission of tuberculosis (Editorial). *JAMA* 280(19):1702–1703.

Barnes PF, Bloch AB, Davidson PT, and Snider DE. 1991. Tuberculosis in patients with human immunodeficiency virus infection. *N Engl J Med* 324:1644–1650.

Barnes PF, Silva C, and Otaya M. 1996. Testing for human immunodeficiency virus infection in patients with tuberculosis. *Am J Respir Crit Care Med* 153:1488–1450.

Barnes PF, Yang Z, Preston-Martin S, et al. 1997. Patterns of tuberculosis transmission in central Los Angeles. *JAMA* 278(14):1159–1163.

Behr MA, Warren SA, Salamon H, Hopewell PC, Ponce de Leon A, Daley CL, and Small PM. 1999. Transmission of *Mycobacterium tuberculosis* from patients smear-negative for acid-fast bacilli. *Lancet* 353:444–449.

Binkin NJ, Vernon AA, Simone PM, et al. 1999. Tuberculosis prevention and control activities in the United States: An overview of the organization of tuberculosis services. *Int J Tuberc Lung Dis* 3(8):663–674.

Binkin NJ, Zuber PLF, Wells CD, Tipple MA, and Castro KG. 1996. Overseas screening for tuberculosis in immigrants and refugees to the United States: Current status. *Clin Infect Dis* 23:1226–1232.

Bishai WR, Graham NM, Harrington S, et al. 1998. Molecular and geographic patterns of tuberculosis transmission after 15 years of directly observed therapy. *JAMA* 280:1679–1684.

Bock NN, Mallory JP, Mobley N, DeVoe B, Brooks Taylor B. 1998. Outbreak of tuberculosis associated with a floating card game in the rural south: Lessons for tuberculosis contact investigations. *Clin Infect Dis* 27:1221–1226.

Booysen C, Van Rie A, Warren R, et al. 1999. The Importance of Contact in the Transmission of Tuberculosis, abstr. 600-PD, p. S37. In: *Proceedings of the IUATLD Meeting in Madrid.* Paris: International Union Against Tuberculosis and Lung Disease.

Brassard P, and Lamarre V. 1999. Evaluation of Tuberculosis Transmission in an Outpatient Pediatric Setting, abstr. 247-PD, p. S188–189. In: *Proceedings of the IUATLD Meeting in Madrid.* Paris: International Union Against Tuberculosis and Lung Disease.

Brook N, Brooks M, Redden D, et al. 1999. A Computer-Based System for TB Contact Investigation. In: *Abstracts of the 1999 ALA/ATS International Conference* in San Diego, California.

Casanova MC, Gonzalez MC, Perez MM, Piqueras AR, Estelles DC, and Morera LM. 1991. The investigation of contacts of the tuberculous pediatric patient. *Med Clin* 97(13):486–490.

Catlos EK, Cantwell MF, Bhatia G, Gedin S, Lewis J, and Mohle-Boetani JC 1998. Public health interventions to encourage TB class A/B1/B2 immigrants to present for TB screening. *Am J Respir Crit Care Med* 158:1037–1041.

California Department of Health Services/California Tuberculosis Controllers Association (CDHS/CTCA). 1998. Joint Guidelines: Contact investigation 1–45.

Cegielski JP, Robison VS, Robinson C, McGaha P, Hassell W, Clark SC. 1997. Community-based screening and prevention of tuberculosis in high risk neighborhoods identified with a geographic information system. In: Program and abstracts of the 37th Interscience Conference on Antimicrobial Agents and Chemotherapy; September 28–October 1, 1997; Toronto, Ontario. Abstract K184:361.

Centers for Disease Control. 1991. Crack cocaine use among persons with tuberculosis—Contra Costa County, California, 1987–1990. *Morbid Mortal Weekly Rep* 40(29):485–489.

Centers for Disease Control. 1987. Multi-drug resistant tuberculosis—North Carolina. *Morbid Mortal Weekly Rep* 35(51–52):785–787.

Centers for Disease Control. 1980. Tuberculosis in a drug rehabilitation center—Colorado. *Morbid Mortal Weekly Rep* 29(45):543–544.

Centers for Disease Control and Prevention. 1999. Tuberculosis elimination revisited: Obstacles, opportunities and renewed commitment. Report of the Advisory Council for the Elimination of Tuberculosis. *Morbid Mortal Weekly Rep* 48(RR-9):1–13.

Centers for Disease Control and Prevention. 1999. Tuberculosis elimination revisited. *Morbid Mortal Weekly Rep* 48(RR-15):1–20.

Centers for Disease Control and Prevention. 1998. Recommendations for prevention and control of TB among foreign-born persons: Report of a Working Group on Tuberculosis among the Foreign Born. *Morbid Mortal Weekly Rep* 47(RR-16):1–30.

Community-based screening and prevention of tuberculosis in high-risk neighborhoods identified with a geographic information system, abstr. K184, p. 361. In: *Program and Abstracts of the 37th Interscience Conference on Antimicrobial Agents and Chemotherapy,* September 28–October 1, 1997. Washington, DC: American Society for Microbiology.

Comstock GW. 1999. How much isoniazid is needed for prevention of tuberculosis among immunocompetent adults? *Int J Tuberc Lung Dis* 10:847–850.

Corless JA, Stockton PA, and Davies PDO. 1999. Is routine screening of all sputum "smear-positive" patients necessary?, abstr. 119-PD, p. S138. In: *Proceedings of the IUATLD meeting in Madrid.* Paris: International Union Against Tuberculosis and Lung Disease.

Daley CL, Small PM, Schecter GF, et al. 1992. An outbreak of tuberculosis with accelerated progression among persons infected with the human immunodeficiency virus. *N Engl J Med* 326:231–235.

Department of Health and Human Services. 1996. *Guide to Clinical Preventive Services,* 2nd Ed. Report of the U.S. Preventive Services Task Force. Washington, DC: DHHS.

DiStasio AJ, and Trump DH. 1990. The investigation of a tuberculosis outbreak in the closed environment of a U.S. Navy ship, 1987. *Military Med* 155(8):347–351.

Ferebee SH. 1970. Controlled chemoprophylaxis trials in tuberculosis: A general review. *Adv Tuberc Res* 17:28–106.

Fernandez RA, Arazo GP, Aguirre EJM, and Arribas LJL. 1994. The study of contacts of tuberculosis patients. *Ann Intern Med* 11(2):62–66.

Fitzpatrick LK, Agerton T, Heirendt W, Valway S, and Onorato I. 1999 Tuberculosis in a small community: A preventable outbreak, abstr. 228-PS, p. S13. In: *Proceedings of the IUATLD Meeting in Madrid.* Paris: International Union Against Tuberculosis and Lung Disease.

Goldman JM, Teale C, Cundall DB, and Pearson SB. 1994. Childhood tuberculosis in Leeds, 1982–90: Social and ethnic factors and the role of the contact clinic in diagnosis. *Thorax* 49(2):184–185.

Greifinger RB, Heywood NJ, and Glaser JB. 1993. Tuberculosis in prison: Balancing justice and public health. *J Law Med Ethics* 21(3–4):332–341.

Hedemark LL. 1996. Contact investigation of a neighborhood bar patron. Investigation of contacts to tuberculosis cases: New York City, June 7–8, 1996. In: *Symposium Summary.* New York: New York City Department of Health.

Holcombe JM. 1996. Contact investigation in a rural setting: A state perspective. Investigation of contacts of tuberculosis cases: New York City, June 7–8, 1996. In: *Symposium Summary.* New York: New York City Department of Health.

Hussain SF, Watura R, Cashman B, Campbell IA, and Evans MR. 1992. Audit of a tuberculosis contact tracing clinic. *Br Med J* 304(6836):1213–1215.

International Union Against Tuberculosis. 1982. Efficacy of various durations of isoniazid preventive therapy for tuberculosis: Five years of follow-up in the IUAT Trial. *Bull WHO* 60(4):555–564.

Iseman MD, 1997. Editorial response: an unholy trinity—Three negative sputum smears and release from tuberculosis isolation. *Clin Infect Dis* 25:671–672.

Jereb JA, Burwen DR, Dooley SW, et al. 1993. Nosocomial outbreak of tuberculosis in a renal transplant unit: Application of a new technique for restriction-fragment-length polymorphism analysis of *Mycobacterium tuberculosis* isolates. *J Infect Dis* 168(5):1219–1224.

Kawamura LM, and Green Rush AM. 1999. TB control tech transfer toolbox: Translating TB control models into step-by-step program guides, abstr. 351-PS, p. S90. In: *Proceedings of the IUATLD Meeting in Madrid*. Paris: International Union Against Tuberculosis and Lung Disease.

Kellogg B, Dye C, Cox K, and Rosenow G. 1987. Public health nursing model for contact follow up of patients with pulmonary tuberculosis. *Public Health Nursing* 4(2):99–104.

Kenyon TA, Ridzon R, Luskin-Hawk R, et al. 1997. A nosocomial outbreak of multidrug-resistant tuberculosis. *Ann Intern Med* 127(1):32–36.

Kenyon TA, Valway SE, Ihle WW, Onorato IM, and Castro KG. 1996. Transmission of multidrug-resistant *Mycobacterium tuberculosis* during a long airplane flight. *N Engl J Med* 334:933–938.

Liippo KK, Kulmala K, and Eero OJT. 1993. Focusing tuberculosis contact tracing by smear grading of index cases. *Am Rev Respir Dis* 148:235–236

Lohuis AMF, van der Werff GFM, Drost AP, Moree C, Vegter B, and Sebek MMGG. 1999. The complete nursing assessment. The development of a standard nursing questionnaire for every patient with TB in The Netherlands, abstr. 136-PS, p. S94. In: *Proceedings of the IUATLD Meeting in Madrid*. Paris: International Union Against Tuberculosis and Lung Disease.

Mangura BT, Napolitano EC, Passannante MR, McDonald RJ, and Reichman LB. 1998. *Mycobacterium tuberculosis* miniepidemic in a church gospel choir. *Chest* 113:234–237.

Marks S, Taylor Z, Nguyen C, Qualls N, Shrestha-Kuwahara R, and Wilce M. 1999. Outcomes of a CDC TB Contact Investigation Study. Preliminary results presented to the Institute of Medicine Committee on the Elimination of Tuberculosis in the United States.

Mehta JB, and Bentley S. 1992. Prevention of tuberculosis in children: Missed opportunities. *Am J Prev Med* 8(5):283–286.

Menzies D. 1997a. Effect of treatment on contagiousness of patients with active tuberculosis. *Infect Control Hosp Epidemiol* 18:582–586.

Menzies D. 1997b. Issues in the management of contacts of patients with active tuberculosis. *Can J Public Health* 88(3):197–201.

Menzies R. 1996. Interpreting contact investigation results: The effect of BCG vaccination. Investigation of contacts to tuberculosis cases: New York City, June 7–8, 1996. In: *Symposium Summary*. New York: New York City Department of Health.

Menzies R, Rocher I, and Vissandjee B. 1993. Factors associated with compliance in treatment of tuberculosis. *Tubercle Lung Dis* 74(1):32–37.

Moodie AS, and Riley RL. 1974. Infectivity of patients with pulmonary tuberculosis in inner city homes. *Am Rev Respir Dis* 110:810–812.

Moore M, Schulte J, Valway SE, et al. 1998. Evaluation of transmission of *Mycobacterium tuberculosis* in a pediatric setting. *J Pediatr* 133:108–112.

Nardell E, Keegan J, Cheney S, and Etkind S. 1991. Airborne infection: Theoretical limits of protection achievable by building ventilation. *Am Rev Respir Dis* 144:302–306.

Nivin B, Nicholas P, Gayer M, Frieden TR, and Fujiwara PI. 1998. A continuing outbreak of multidrug-resistant tuberculosis, with transmission in a hospital nursery. *Clin Infect Dis* 26:303–307.

Nolan CM, Goldberg SV, and Buskin SE. 1999. Hepatoxicity associated with isoniazid preventive therapy: A seven-year survey from a public health tuberculosis clinic. *JAMA* 281:1014–1018.

Onorato I. 1999. Managing TB Outbreaks. Centers for Disease Control and Prevention presentation to the Institute of Medicine Committee on the Elimination of Tuberculosis in the United States.

Peerbooms PGH, van Doornum GJJ, van Deutekom H, Coutinho RA, and van Soolingen D. 1995. Laboratory-acquired tuberculosis. *Lancet* 345:1311–1312.

Pena A, Anibarro L, Sanjurjp A, Nunes MJ, Garcia JC, and Romay A. 1999. Childhood transmission of tuberculosis, abstr. 561-PD, p. S192. In: *Proceedings of the IUATLD Meeting in Madrid*. Paris: International Union Against Tuberculosis and Lung Disease.

Rodriguez EM, Steinbart S, Shaulis G, Bur S, and Dwyer DM. 1996. Pulmonary tuberculosis in a high school student and a broad contact investigation: Lessons relearned. *Md Med J* 45(12):1019–1022.

Rothenburg RB. 1996. Social network approach in contact tracing. Investigation of Contacts to tuberculosis cases: New York City, June 7–8, 1996. In: *Symposium Summary*. New York: New York City Department of Health.

Rubilar M, Brochwicz-Lewinski MJ, Anderson M, and Leitch AG. 1995. The outcome of contact procedures for tuberculosis in Edinburgh, Scotland, 1982–1991. *Respir Med* 89(2):113–120.

Rubin FL, and Lynch DC. 1996. Tuberculosis control through contact investigation. *Penn Med* 22–23.

Sasaki Y, Yamagishi F, and Suzuki K. 1995. The present condition of patient's, doctor's and total delays in tuberculosis case finding and countermeasures in the future *Kekkaku* 70(1):49–55.

Shrestha-Kuwahara R, Wilce M, Deluca N, Rosenbaum J, and Taylor Z. 1999. Patient provider communication during TB contact investigation, abstr. 219-PD, p. S139. In: *Proceedings of the IUATLD Meeting in Madrid*. Paris: International Union Against Tuberculosis and Lung Disease.

Snider DE, Kelly GD, Cauthen GM, Thompson NJ, and Kilburn JO. 1985. Infection and disease among contacts of tuberculosis cases with drug-resistant and drug-susceptible bacilli. *Am Rev Respir Dis* 132:125–132.

Tabet SR, Goldbaum GM, Hooton TM, Eisenach KD, Cave MD, and Nolan CM. 1994. Restriction-fragment-length polymorphism analysis detecting a community-based outbreak among persons infected with human immunodeficiency virus. *J Infect Dis* 169:189–192

Topley JM, Maher D, and Mbewe LN. 1996. Transmission of tuberculosis to contacts of sputum-positive adults in Malawi. *Arch Dis Child* 74(2):140–143.

Valway SE, Sanchez MPC, Shinnick TF, et al. 1998. An outbreak involving extensive transmission of a virulent strain of *Mycobacterium tuberculosis*. *N Engl J Med* 338(10):633–639.

van Soolingen D, Lambregts-van Weezenbeek CSB, de Haas PEW, Veen J, and van Embden JDA. 1996. Transmission of sensitive and resistant strains of *Mycobacterium tuberculosis* in The Netherlands, 1993–1995. *Nederlands Tijdschr Geneesk* 140:2286–2289.

Veening GJ. 1968. Long-term isoniazid prophylaxis: Controlled trial on INH prophylaxis after recent tuberculin conversion in young adults. *Bull Int Union Tuberc* 41:169–171.

Washko R, Robinson E, Fehrs LJ, and Frieden TR. 1998. Tuberculosis transmission in a high school choir. *J School Health* 68(6):256–259.

Wells CD, Zuber PLF, Nolan CM Binkin NJ, and Goldberg SV. 1997. Tuberculosis prevention among foreign-born persons in Seattle-King County, Washington. *Am J Respir Crit Care Med* 156:573–577.

Zhang Y, Heym B, Allen B, Young D, and Cole S. 1992. The catalase-peroxidase gene and isoniazid resistance of *Mycobacterium tuberculosis*. *Nature* 358:591–593.

5

Developing the Tools for Tuberculosis Elimination

At the current rate of decline, approximately 6 percent per year, it will take more than 70 years to reach the target for elimination of tuberculosis of 1 case of tuberculosis per million population. Even if the rate of decline is accelerated to 10 percent per year it will take about 50 years to reach the target. New tools are clearly needed to accelerate the rate of decline to one at which elimination becomes a realistic objective in the next 2 or 3 decades. A great deal of attention has been focused on the development of a new vaccine for the prevention of tuberculosis infection. However, because so many of the cases in the United States are not the result of recent transmission of tuberculosis but rather are the result of reactivation of latent infection, the greatest needs in the United States are new diagnostic tools for the more accurate identification of individuals who are truly infected and who are also at risk of developing tuberculosis. Together with new treatments—drugs or immunological adjuvants—for the prevention of disease in infected individuals, that are easily administered, the elimination of tuberculosis can be a reality. New drugs will also be needed for the treatment of disease both to overcome multidrug resistant strains of tuberculosis and to shorten and simplify current treatment regimens. As all of these new tools will likely contribute to the global fight against tuberculosis, their applicabilities need to be studied. This chapter reviews the current tuberculosis research efforts and outlines strategies for improvement.

RECOMMENDATIONS

Recommendation 5.1 To advance the development of tuberculosis vaccines the committee recommends that the plans outlined in the *Blueprint for Tuberculosis Vaccine Development*, published by the National Institutes of Health (NIH) in 1998, be fully implemented.

Recommendation 5.2 To advance the development of diagnostic tests and new drugs for both latent infection and active disease, action plans should be developed and implemented. The Centers for Disease Control and Prevention (CDC) should then exploit its expertise in population-based research to evaluate and define the role of promising products.

Recommendation 5.3 To promote better understanding of patient and provider nonadherence with tuberculosis recommendations and guidelines a plan for a behavioral and social science research agenda should be developed and implemented.

Recommendation 5.4 To encourage private-sector product development, the global market for tuberculosis diagnostic tests, drugs, and vaccines should be better characterized and access to these markets for these new products should be facilitated.

Recommendation 5.5 To define the applicability of any new tools to the international arena and facilitate their development, the U.S. Agency for International Development (AID), NIH, and CDC should build upon international relationships and expertise to conduct research.

BACKGROUND AND INTRODUCTION

In 1989, the CDC Advisory Council for the Elimination of Tuberculosis (ACET) called for the development and evaluation of new technologies for tuberculosis diagnosis, treatment, and prevention and the rapid transfer of newly developed technologies into clinical and public health practice. The International Task Force echoed this sentiment for disease eradication and concluded in 1993 (Centers for Disease Control and Prevention, 1993) that tuberculosis could not be eradicated without better tests, treatments, case findings, and vaccines. In the years that have passed since these pronouncements, progress has been made on all of these fronts, but much remains to be done. This chapter reviews the current status and needs for tuberculosis diagnosis, treatment, and prevention, the dynamics that influence research efforts, and the ongoing activities of the key groups involved. It also identifies the research efforts needed to accelerate the decline in cases and the move toward the elimination of tuberculosis.

CURRENT STATUS AND NEEDS

Diagnostic Methods

Currently, the management of tuberculosis is dependent on the ability to identify individuals with active disease, those whose disease is caused by organisms resistant to antimicrobial agents, those who are infected but not ill, and those who are most likely to progress from infection to disease. Although precise numbers are not known, the World Health Organization (WHO) (Mark Perkins, personal communication) estimates that each year sputum examiners screen approximately 60 million to 80 million people for active tuberculosis and that multiple examinations are conducted for each of these people. However, even gross estimates of the number of tuberculin skin tests, for acid-fast bacilli (AFB) smears, radiographs, cultures, or other tests are not available. Although great strides have been made in decreasing the burden of tuberculosis in the United States by using existing technologies, there is considerable room for improvement in each of these endeavors, particularly in children, human immunodeficiency virus (HIV)-infected individuals, and the increasing numbers of patients with tuberculosis outside of their lungs.

The microscopic examination of sputa for the detection of AFB (AFB smear) is rapid, technically simple, and widely available and identifies those thought to be most infectious to others. However, WHO estimates that AFB is identified by sputum microscopy in only 35 percent of people with active tuberculosis (Raviglione et al., 1997). Furthermore, a molecular epidemiological approach has demonstrated that even in efficiently administered tuberculosis control programs, those persons who are AFB smear negative account for at least 15 percent of cases of disease transmission (Behr et al., 1999). Laboratory techniques for the replacement or improvement of the detection of AFB in clinical specimens that address these limitations would greatly enhance patient care and infection control.

Cultivation of mycobacteria from specimens obtained from persons suspected of having tuberculosis remains the mainstay for the diagnosis of tuberculosis and the identification of bacterial strains that are resistant to antibiotics. The use of rapid radiometric techniques has greatly decreased the time required for cultivation and susceptibility testing of mycobacteria, and the use of DNA probes can speed the identification of organisms once they are growing in culture (Crawford, 1994). However, these techniques still require an average of 10 to 14 days and are generally available only in reference laboratories. The delay in reporting because specimens are being evaluated through a cascade of different laboratories can be long.

Nucleic acid amplification tests for the direct detection of *Mycobacterium tuberculosis* in clinical specimens remain one of the unfulfilled promises in tuberculosis. Eagerly anticipated nucleic amplification assays that can detect the presence of *M. tuberculosis* in hours, such as the polymerase chain reaction (PCR), are now licensed. However, the fact that uncertainties remain about the appropriate use of such techniques in clinical practice, despite numerous peer-reviewed publications on this topic, illustrates the challenges in assessing the strengths and limitations of new diagnostic methods and defining their appropriate role in the context of classic diagnostic algorithms and diverse clinical settings (Anonymous, 1997). This vast yet inadequate literature demonstrates the manner in which a lack of coordination between basic scientists and industry can yield an obstructed pipeline of product development. Defining the rational use of existing tests and streamlining the evaluation of new tests are clear and present needs.

Over the past decade, bacterial genotyping techniques have become routine for the identification and tracking of individual strains and have greatly enhanced the ability to detect point source outbreaks and laboratory cross-contamination. However, a demonstrable impact of these on disease control is lacking. If molecular biological methods could be developed for the identification of specific strains that are highly transmissible or that have an enhanced capacity to cause progression to active disease in the host, public health officials could more efficiently focus efforts on contact identification and treatment of latent infection.

In contrast to recent advances in clinical mycobacteriology, there have been no improvements in the ability to identify persons who are latently infected with *M. tuberculosis*. Tuberculin skin testing with purified protein derivatives from *M. tuberculosis* has remained essentially unchanged for more than 60 years. This test requires trained personnel for administration and interpretation, two patient encounters within 2 to 7 days, and is falsely negative for approximately 20 percent of individuals with active disease and a greater percentage of the growing numbers of persons coinfected with HIV (Holden et al., 1971; Nunn and Douglas, 1980). Because of cross-reactivity with mycobacteria other than *M. tuberculosis* and *Mycobacterium bovis*, complex algorithms of different clinical cutoff points continue to confuse health care providers (Huebner et al., 1993). New reagents or assays are needed to address these limitations (Streeton et al., 1988). Whole genome approaches provide the promise of identifying species-specific antigens, but exploitation of this approach and validation of new tests will be methodologically and logistically challenging.

Rational targeting of treatment to those individuals infected with *M. tuberculosis* is hampered by the inability to reliably predict who among them will progress to active disease. Although the clinical and epidemiological characteristics of patients likely to progress to active disease (such as silicosis, diabetes, injection drug use, and low weight) have been discussed for decades, the majority of individuals who do progress to active disease lack these characteristics. Thus, the current proposal is the treatment of all individuals identified to have latent infection, even though active infection will be reactivated in only 10 percent or less of these individuals. Evidence of host genetic factors and surrogate markers of protection would permit targeted interventions.

A new method for the diagnosis of latent infection should be highly specific and ideally will identify those individuals who harbor viable tubercle bacilli or who are at risk for active tuberculosis in the future. In Chapter 4, selective skin testing by country of origin based on the prevalence of infected individuals in that country is suggested. A more specific test would permit a more broad-based screening as the possibility of false-positive reactions is reduced. However, even among those who are most recently infected and disease-free, only 10 to 15 percent will develop disease in the future. The ability to distinguish that group from those who have developed an immune response that will prevent the development of disease will greatly enhance the efficiency of any effort to prevent disease among latently infected individuals. Even with the regimens currently available for the treatment of latent infection, a highly specific test that detects individuals at the highest risk of developing disease in the future would have a greater impact on the elimination of tuberculosis in the United States than a vaccine that prevents infection. Such a test might also make the treatment of latent infection in many countries with medium and low average incomes a practical intervention.

Drugs

Once identified, persons who are either ill from *M. tuberculosis* infection or infected with *M. tuberculosis* can be treated with a high degree of success. However, current approaches to the treatment of tuberculosis have serious limitations. Treatment of tuberculosis currently requires the administration of multiple different agents for a minimum of 6 months. Success in the treatment of disease in the growing number of persons with disease caused by strains of *M. tuberculosis* resistant to antibiotics is less certain, requiring a considerably longer duration of therapy and considerable toxicity. The treatment of asymptomatic tuberculosis infection with potentially toxic drugs is based on an algorithm so complex as to be misunderstood by most health care providers and thus is often applied to less than half of the eligible individuals.

Since streptomycin, the drug first effective in the treatment of tuberculosis, was released and approved for general clinical study and use in 1948, a number of other antimicrobial agents have been approved for use in this disease (See Table 1 in Appendix F). Decades of coordinated clinical trials have demonstrated that these agents can be used in a dizzying number of regimens (Iseman and Sbarbaro, 1991). However, treatment of tuberculosis still requires the simultaneous administration of multiple different drugs for protracted periods. Given the pharmacokinetics of agents approved for use in the United States, most of these drugs require frequent dosing, and cure of tuberculosis now requires that a patient consume a minimum of seven tablets each day.

Unfortunately, these established treatment regimens are increasingly ineffective because of the increasing incidence of tuberculosis due to drug-resistant *M. tuberculosis* in the United States and around the world. For example, in a survey of *M. tuberculosis* isolates obtained from 13,511 patients in the United States between 1994 and 1997, 12.3 percent had drug resistance among newly diagnosed and previously untreated patients to any (isoniazid, rifampin, streptomycin, ethambutol) drug, 8.2 percent had primary resistance to one drug, and 4.1 percent had primary resistance to more than one drug (Pablos-Méndez et al., 1998). In the same survey the prevalence of drug resistance among an additional 833 isolates from previously treated individuals in the United States was considerably higher: 23.6 percent were resistant to any drug, 12.5 percent were resistant to one drug (8.1 percent were resistant to isoniazid), 11.2 percent were resistant to more than one drug, and 2.0 percent were resistant to four drugs. Problems of drug resistance are considerably greater in other parts of the world. For example, among isolates from 575 patients in Latvia, 41.6 percent were resistant (combined primary and acquired) to any drug, 34.7 percent were resistant to more than one drug, and 7.0 percent were resistant to all four drugs (Pablos-Méndez et al., 1998). There are limited data on treatment outcomes for subsets of patients with specific single-drug resistance.

Most troubling is the emergence of multidrug-resistant strains that are resistant to at least the two most powerful drugs, isoniazid and rifampin. In contrast to single-drug-resistant strains, which can be effectively treated with prolonged courses of alternative drugs, the success of treatment of multidrug-resistant tuberculosis is only marginally better than outcomes of tuberculosis in the prechemotherapy era. In a report on global surveillance for antituberculosis drug resistance, the data for the United States indicated that the combined rates of primary and acquired multidrug resistance was 2.0 percent (Pablos-Méndez et al., 1998). In India, a country which accounts for about 30,000 immigrants to the United States each year, multidrug-resistant isolates occurred in 13.3 percent of patients. Closer to the United States, data from Mexico suggest multidrug resistance rates of 6 percent (Centers for Disease Control, 1998). More recent data, however, suggest that the early diagnosis and treatment of tuberculosis have resulted in improved outcomes for patients with tuberculosis in Mexico.

The need for both shorter, simpler, and less toxic regimens and regimens for the treatment of disease caused by multidrug-resistant *M. tuberculosis* provides ample cause for the development of new agents. However, the development of new antituberculosis drugs by pharmaceutical companies in recent decades has faltered and has fallen behind that of other antimicrobial agents, to a large extent because of the perceived relatively limited market of patients with active tuberculosis in the United States (19,851 cases in 1997). During the 5-year period between 1992 and 1996, a total of 42 new antimicrobial drugs (exclusive of topical agents, additional indications for older drugs, and new preparations of older drugs for different routes of administration) were approved by the U.S. Food and Drug Administration (FDA). Of the 42 new antimicrobial drugs, 17 were antibacterial drugs, 14 were antiviral agents;, 4 were antifungal drugs, 5 were antiparasitic drugs, and only 2 were antituberculosis drugs. Indeed, of the latter two drugs, only one, rifabutin, a drug in the rifamycin group (like rifampin), was a new drug; the other was rifater, a combination of three already long-approved drugs (isoniazid, pyrazinamide, and rifampin). Another drug, levofloxacin (the more active isomer of ofloxacin), active against *M. tuberculosis*, was approved for use as an antibacterial agent, not for the primary treatment of tuberculosis. Another new rifamycin group drug, rifapentine, was approved by FDA in 1998 for the treatment of pulmonary tuberculosis. Its principal difference from rifampin is in its pharmacokinetics (half-life of 13.2 hours, versus a half-life of 3.4 hours for rifampin), allowing twice-weekly dosing during the 2-month intensive dosing phase of multidrug treatment and once-weekly dosing in the four-month continuation phase of the short-course program of therapy. In sum, in the past 7-year period, no fundamentally new antituberculosis drugs have been approved for the treatment of either tuberculosis infection or multidrug-resistant tuberculosis.

Significant advances have been made in understanding the mechanisms by which *M. tuberculosis* resists antimicrobial agents, but the mechanisms remain to be defined for many agents. Furthermore, none of these insights have been translated into tangible improvements in clinical practice.

Options for the treatment of tuberculosis infection, although recently expanded (American Thoracic Society, 2000) remain problematic. Isoniazid, the drug for which the most data are available, requires at least 9 months of daily therapy to be maximally effective. Although recently approved, the combination of rifampin and pyrazinamide for 2 months is based on limited data. There are even fewer scientific data for a 4-month course of rifampin. Prospects for new drugs for the treatment of latent infection are hampered by the lack of techniques for the screening of drug activity against latent bacteria. In combination with increasing rates of drug-resistant tuberculosis, treatment of tuberculosis infection is particularly problematic. It has been inferred, although never rigorously documented, that resistance to isoniazid negates the efficacy of treatment of latent infection with isoniazid. Similarly, newer regimens with rifampin and pyrazinamide are likely to be relatively ineffective against multidrugresistant strains.

Even when effective regimens are available for the treatment of infections caused by drug-resistant organisms, it is unclear how regimens will be selected for individual patients since it is generally impossible to know the susceptibility of the latent bacilli that they harbor. A lack of understanding of immunity hampers efforts to develop immunomodulators, although thalidomide is a promising proof of principle for the concept of immune modulator in tuberculosis treatment.

Vaccines

The only available vaccine against tuberculosis is BCG, originally developed by Calmette and Guérin by attenuation through serial passage of an *M. bovis* strain 230 times in vitro between 1908 and 1921. The protective efficacy rates of this vaccine have varied widely when studied over the past half century. Controlled trials and case-control trials have shown protective efficacy rates of the vaccine have a wide range from less than zero percent (i.e., vaccinated individuals were at higher risk) to 75 to 80 percent (Centers for Disease Control and Prevention, 1996). Postulated reasons for this variability include differences in the rate of background infection with environmental mycobacteria, differences in vaccine strains that developed before seed lots were stabilized in a lyophilized form, and other factors related to the patient's environment and socioeconomic status. Two meta-analyses (10 randomized clinical trials and 8 case-control studies in one meta-analysis and 14 clinical trials and 12 case control trials in the second one) have been performed and indicate that the efficacy of the BCG vaccine against meningeal and miliary tuberculosis in children was high (i.e., 80 to 85 percent), but the efficacy of the vaccine against pulmonary tuberculosis differed markedly between the studies of the first meta-analysis and was sufficiently wide as to preclude determination of a summary protective efficacy rate (Rodrigues et al., 1993). In the second meta-analysis the overall protective efficacy of BCG was calculated as 50 percent (Colditz et al., 1994). When present, the efficacy of vaccination with the BCG vaccine has been shown to persist for at least 10 years (Sterne et al., 1998) and may last for more than 20 years (Aronson et al., 1999).

Much has been written that describes the attributes of an ideal tuberculosis vaccine. The list includes safety and the ability to protect against infection and disease, be easily administered, be long-lasting, be inexpensive, be heat stable, not interfere with tuberculin skin testing, and be easily integrated into existing immunization schedules. A less well explored topic is the mechanism by which candidate vaccines can be evaluated for these variables. The difficulty in conducting clinical trials with vaccines against tuberculosis is exemplified by the fact that many of these attributes remain controversial for BCG after more than 70 years of clinical experience. Given the unlikelihood of identifying a perfect tuberculosis vaccine in the proximate future, it is important to define what would comprise a minimally acceptable vaccine or combination of vaccines to meet global needs.

The needs for and approach to tuberculosis vaccine development were recently elucidated at a workshop convened by the U.S. Department of Health and Human Services, the U.S. National Vaccine Program Office, and NIH (National Institutes of Health, 1998). This workshop emphasized the need for a coordinated, multifaceted, minimal, long-term commitment of $800 million over the coming 20 years. Initial steps proposed a focus on basic research, animal models, clinical trial design, and international capacity building. These will need to be linked to vaccine production facilities and epidemiologically well-characterized U.S. and international field sites.

Operational

The WHO Global Tuberculosis Research Initiative has identified social science research as a priority. Earlier a call for a similar agenda had been made in the United States (Centers for Disease Control and Prevention, 1995).

Despite the renewed focus on tuberculosis in the United States, many health care providers remain ignorant about tuberculosis, many health care systems do not prioritize it, and many patients do not adhere to the treatment. Thus, there is a need to understand the determinants of behavior of health care providers and systems (e.g., health maintenance organizations) as well as the behavior of patients and to improve methods for predicting and monitoring patient adherence and compliance with therapy, particularly in marginalized populations and immigrants. A panel of effective methods that can be used to enhance patient and provider adherence and compliance must be developed and implemented in a targeted fashion. The need to understand the determinants of behavior is particularly acute for the development of programs for the treatment of latent infection. Asking people to take medication for a disease that they do not yet have is likely to present a totally new set of challenges. In addition, the call for programs of treatment for latent infection among foreign-born individuals presents yet another dimension of the need to understand human behavior, as ethnic variations in knowledge, attitudes, and behavior need to be elucidated and understood. There has been a recent effort to understand the costs and economics of tuberculosis, especially through the Prevention Effectiveness Studies Section, in the Research Branch of the Division of Tuberculosis Elimination. This research needs to be expanded and will be central to selecting the most cost-effective strategies as incidence declines. Another area for operational research, contact investigations and outbreaks, is described in Chapter 4.

DYNAMICS OF TUBERCULOSIS RESEARCH

An evaluation of current and future research activities must recognize and account for the different goals, expertise, priority-setting mechanisms, and evaluation criteria of the diverse partners in tuberculosis research. Such an understanding both will explain current activities and is crucial in any attempt to influence the focus of these efforts. The ultimate goal of implementing an efficient pipeline of research from the "bench to the bedside" can be met by recognizing and influencing these dynamics. These partners can be broadly classified as basic, applied, and operational researchers.

The goal of basic investigators is to advance fundamental knowledge in the biology of tuberculosis. This goal is pursued by highly specialized individuals who are largely working in academic and research institutes using a broad array of modern techniques that have been developed in diverse scientific fields such as bacteriology and immunology. In general, the focus of their efforts is set by individual investigators' perceptions of the importance and opportunities in their fields. The actual research portfolio is heavily influenced by the availability of research funds, as demonstrated by the dramatic expansion of basic tuberculosis research efforts stimulated by recent increases in funding for such research. These investigations are largely evaluated by peer review of grant applications and the publications that result from the research.

Applied researchers aim to translate basic knowledge into pragmatic applications. These efforts can be further dichotomized into early "proof-of-principle" efforts (largely conducted by investigators in academia and the biotechnology industry) and developmental efforts (almost exclusively conducted by workers in the pharmaceutical and diagnostics industries). As such, although these individuals' priorities are influenced by the availability of public research funds, they are primarily influenced by industrial decision makers on the basis of the perceived economics of the potential market. Their productivity can be evaluated in terms of the patents and products that are ultimately marketed.

The goal of operational researchers is to optimize the efficiency of application of licensed technologies. Thus, operational researchers require an understanding of the realities of the situations in which tuberculosis is being diagnosed (such as the factors that influence health care providers and clients) and an ability to work effectively in partnership with these communities. The major contributors in these efforts are the CDC, WHO, and a small number of academic investigators and members of nongovernmental organizations. Priorities in this realm are set by the potential of their efforts to affect outcomes. As such, they are evaluated by the policies that they establish and ultimately by the effects that these policies have on clinical outcomes.

CURRENT ACTIVITIES

National Institutes of Health (NIH)

In 1989, a year in which more than 2 million people died from tuberculosis, only a few NIH-funded laboratories were investigating *M. tuberculosis*. Largely in response to the resurgence of the disease in the United States, the early 1990s was a time of unprecedented expansion in NIH-sponsored tuberculosis research (Figure 5-1).

By 1995, the total NIH budget for tuberculosis research was $62 million. This expansion has been followed by a period of stagnation, in which funding for tuberculosis research increased only slightly faster than the overall rate of inflation. The vast majority of this research funding is administered by the National Institute of Allergy and Infectious Diseases ($41.7 million), and the National Heart, Lung, and Blood Institute ($16.1 million), but also includes the National Institute of Drug Abuse ($6.6 million), the National Center for Research Resources ($4.8 million), Fogarty International Center ($2.2 million), National Institute of Diabetes and Digestive and Kidney Diseases ($1.5 million), National Institute of Child Health and Human Development ($0.8 million), National Institute on Alcohol Abuse and Alcoholism ($0.5 million), National Institute of Mental Health ($0.4 million), and the National Institute of Nursing Research ($0.4 million).

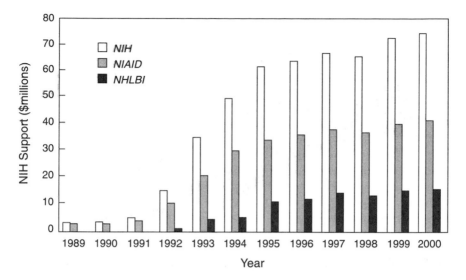

FIGURE 5-1 National Institutes of Health support of tuberculosis research. SOURCE: National Institutes of Health.

The research sponsored by NIH can be classified into U.S. Public Health Service categories of pathogenesis, diagnostics, therapeutics, vaccines, epidemiology, and training. Data on funding for tuberculosis research from the National Institute of Allergy and Infectious Diseases are presented in Figure 5-2.

Although most of this work is extramural, with the $35 million award to the Tuberculosis Research Unit being the largest single extramural award, three intramural research programs focus on tuberculosis. The majority of the extramural research is funded through investigator-initiated research grants. In addition, non-hypothesis-driven efforts are funded through contracts focused on three areas: research materials and vaccine testing, a coordinated research unit, and a facility for drug screening.

Training of young scientists in the field of tuberculosis research is a stated priority of NIH and occurs both through programs targeted toward tuberculosis (e.g., the Tuberculosis International Research Training Program) and through generally focused graduate and postdoctoral fellowships. In addition, the National Heart, Lung, and Blood Institute has a specific program targeted toward curriculum development to teach young scientists about tuberculosis.

Although no single parameter accurately assesses the productivity of research, in the realm of basic science, the numbers of papers published

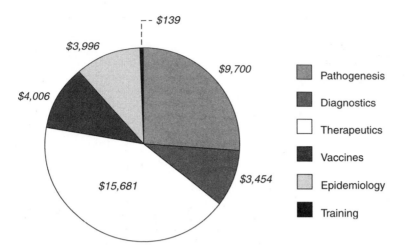

FIGURE 5-2 National Institute of Allergy and Infectious Diseases Fiscal Year 1998 tuberculosis funding by Public Health Service category (in $thousands). SOURCE: National Institutes of Health.

and the number of citations that they receive in other papers or reports is perhaps the best. Figure 5-3 shows the numbers of Medline publications under the heading of "tuberculosis" by year between 1989 and 1998. These publications have been divided according to the 19 relevant MESH sub-headings, which have been grouped into five categories (pathogenesis/ vaccines, diagnostics, therapy/complications, epidemiology/control, and other). Of note, the total number of annual publications, which was roughly stable from 1966 to 1989, increased through the early 1990s as funding and public attention was increasing. Importantly, the types of publications have remained balanced. Thus, from this admittedly imperfect measure, one senses that productivity in tuberculosis research has increased and balance has been maintained in the research portfolio.

Centers for Disease Control and Prevention

The research programs of CDC currently encompass a broad range of activities including basic bacteriological research, surveillance, operational research, behavioral studies, technology assessment, and transfer. Although it is difficult to precisely account for funds spent on these efforts (as opposed to related activities), the total research budget is $15 million per year, approximately 10 percent of the overall CDC budget for tuberculosis.

Among this diverse group of activities, several seem to be particu-

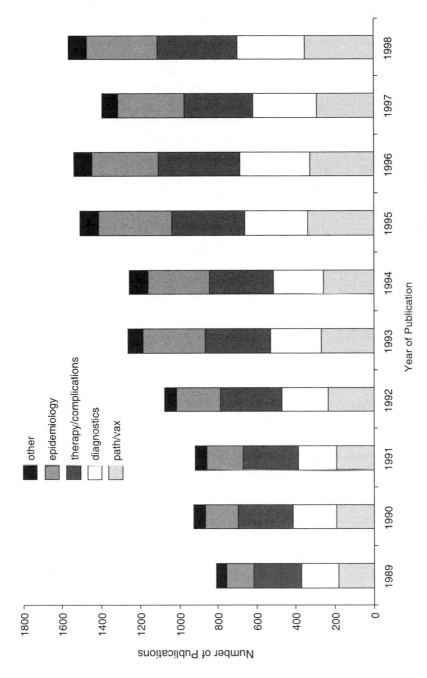

FIGURE 5-3 Number of Medline publications for tuberculosis, by type, per year, 1989 to 1998.

larly productive. CDC surveillance activities (which incorporate novel technologies such as bacterial genotyping) are among the best in the world. Detailed descriptive analysis of disease risk and burden are available and provide a wealth of material for rational improvements in disease control. The Tuberculosis Trials Consortium (TBTC) initiated in 1995 was instrumental in the licensure of rifapentine in 1998. CDC-sponsored clinical trials provided crucial data on which the new recommendations of use of the combination of rifampin and pyrazinamide for the treatment of tuberculous infection were based. CDC has published approximately 20 peer-reviewed papers each year, roughly equally divided among the areas of basic science, diagnostics, and epidemiology.

One apparent impediment to realizing the potential of CDC research is administrative division between epidemiological and laboratory activities. Epidemiological research and control activities are situated in the National Center for HIV, STD, and Tuberculosis Prevention, in the Division of Tuberculosis Elimination, whereas laboratory activities and research are housed in the National Center for Infectious Diseases, in the Division of AIDS, STD, and Tuberculosis Laboratory Research. Although most CDC staff report that communications are good and improving, the perception of many researchers outside of CDC is that there is often a lack of communication and coordination.

New Tuberculosis Diagnostic Developments by Industry

The most systematic assessment of members of industry with an interest in the development of tuberculosis diagnostic tools has been conducted by Mark Perkins, WHO, director of the Tuberculosis Diagnostics Initiative of WHO (personal communication, 1999). They were identified at international meetings, via word of mouth, in response to spontaneous requests for information or referral of such requests from other agencies, through publication of information on the tuberculosis diagnostic initiative, and in discussions with pharmacists and private physicians in developing countries. As of 1999, 58 commercial agencies or academic researchers with industry developmental support have been identified through this survey. Many of the test developers are small diagnostic companies, some of whom had interacted frequently with WHO regarding specimen acquisition, market understanding, and the design of trials for the assessment of diagnostic tools. The respondents had various levels of willingness to share information, spanning a spectrum, from those willing to speak openly about their development plans to others unwilling to discuss even the format of the tools in development or the target matrix. There are many fewer diagnostic approaches than there are industry or academic test developers. This represents both the use by multiple companies of tests with the same type and format (with serological assays that target immunoglobulin directed against a single *M. tuberculosis* antigen being the most common) and the simple repackaging of single products by more than one company. Companies may market diagnostic tools developed in their own facilities (or under contract) as well as those developed by other companies and licensed for marketing under a different name. The reticence of some companies to disclose the nature and development or production site of their products has made it difficult to determine the extent to which the number of companies identified in the survey to be involved with tuberculosis diagnostic tools is inflated by marketing of duplicate products.

Given the limitations in information and the confidentiality agreements under which much of the information was obtained, it is not possible to list the companies identified in the survey of tuberculosis diagnostics, the specifications of the tests that companies are developing, or in some cases even the type of assay being developed. However, Table 5-1 summarizes the range of tests that were found to be under development.

One proxy for potential industrial interest in tuberculosis is the number of U.S. patents filed. Although this clearly reflects activities funded from a variety of sources and conducted by different types of people, it is an objective measure. Figure 5-4 shows the number of tuberculosis-related U.S. patents issued by year as determined by searching the International Business Machines Corp. Intellectual Property Network (http://patent.womplex.ibm.com/). By searching all fields on the U.S. patents front pages, it is possible to observe a dramatic increase in the number of tuberculosis-related patents issued over time.

TABLE 5-1 Number of Companies Developing Tests for Diagnosis of Tuberculosis by Type of Test

Type of Test	Number of Companies
Undisclosed	16
Antibody production	15
Nucleic acid amplification	10
Cellular immune response	5
Novel culture method	4
Antigen detection	4
Phage selection	2
Chemical detection	2

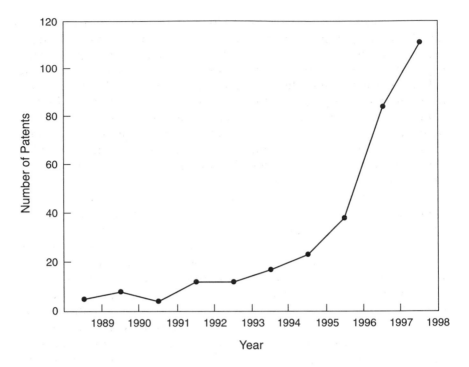

FIGURE 5-4 Number of U.S. tuberculosis patents for tuberculosis diagnostic tools, 1989 to 1998.

New Drug Development by Industry

To determine the current activity in the biotechnology and pharmaceutical industries in the field of new drug discovery, the committee has explored two questions: (1) Has industry reported new lead compounds or drugs in the antimicrobial literature? (2) Are biotechnology and pharmaceutical companies pursuing new drugs that are still in initial phases of development? To answer the first question the committee searched by title for articles that dealt with new antimicrobial agents and that were published in three 2-year periods (1988–1989, 1992–1993, and 1997–1998) in *Antimicrobial Agents and Chemotherapy*, the leading U.S. journal that deals with new anti-infective drugs. During the aforementioned periods, a total of 374 new (not previously reported) drugs were noted in the titles of 374 articles. Forty percent described antibacterial drugs, 20 percent described antiviral agents, but only 3 percent described antimycobacterial agents. When drugs with primary activity against only *Mycobacterium leprae* or *Mycobacterium avium* complex are eliminated, only eight drugs remain, of which two are rifabutin and ofloxacin, and the remainder represent only 1.7 percent of the total.

To answer the second question 22 major pharmaceutical companies and 7 biotechnology companies (see Table 2 and Table 3 in Appendix F) were contacted by phone and asked if they had any new drugs in the pipeline that might be forthcoming in the next 2, 5, or 8 years for use in the treatment of tuberculosis. The results are quite discouraging regarding current discovery efforts. Only four companies indicated that they had any drugs in the pipeline for the time frame as mentioned above. Only one company noted that it had oxazolidinone compounds undergoing preliminary laboratory investigation and, if results were encouraging, would require 5 to 8 years before they might become available for clinical use (Cynamon et al., 1999). Another company noted that it had oxazolidinone compounds undergoing preliminary laboratory investigation, but it had turned over its rights to develop the drug to the company mentioned in the previous sentence. A third company noted that it has no track record with the development of antituberculosis drugs but had found a group of compounds in an antibacterial screening process that it is sending elsewhere for in vitro testing. The marketing team at this company is unenthusiastic about pursuing such a drug(s) because of the limited U.S. market. Finally, one major pharmaceutical company was recently involved in preliminary work with animals on the use of interleukin 12 (IL-12) as an interferon inducer on the basis of the known actions of IL-12. However, the work was recently abandoned when it was found in an experimental animal model of *M. tuberculosis* infection that treatment with this biological response modifier paradoxically increased the number of *M. tuberculosis* bacilli in the lungs.

Among the seven biotechnology companies that the committee contacted, one is pursuing development of a nitroimidizopyrene, which inhibits glycolipid cell wall synthesis (at a step different than that at which it is inhibited by ethambutol). It appears to be bactericidal and active against both replicating and nongrowing organisms. If all goes well with future testing, the company believes that the drug might be available for clinical use in 5 to 8 years. The same company has also been developing a rifamycin analog (rifalizyl) with a longer half-life, but the company is giving up development of this analog because *M. tuberculosis* strains resistant to rifampin show cross-resistance to it. Another biotechnology company is working on three candidate ethambutol analogs that should be ready for clinical testing in the next 2 to 5 years. Another candidate drug, one that inhibits the shikemic acid pathway, is in the preliminary testing phase and is 5 to 8 years away from possible clinical use. Finally, one company is studying the use of a combination of IL-12 plus three conventional antituberculosis drugs for the treatment of *M. tuberculosis or M.*

avium-M. intracellulare infection in patients with AIDS. The same company is involved in a current clinical study of the combination of IL-12 plus three conventional antituberculosis drugs for the treatment of tuberculosis in The Gambia. Neither study, if the results prove positive, is expected to lead to clinical use of the drugs before 5 to 8 years hence. It should be noted that this approach involves the auxiliary use of a biological response modifier rather than a new antimicrobial agent.

The cost of drug development and the lack of a market for antituberculosis drugs are often cited as barriers to the development of new drugs for the treatment of tuberculosis. The commonly cited cost for the development of a new drug is $350 million. Even if this estimate is accurate it amortizes the cost of all failed candidate drugs into the cost of the successful drug. This is not a legitimate estimate for an antituberculosis drug, given the amount of public funding that supports drug research. This support not only includes the type of basic research commonly associated with NIH but also includes programs to provide rapid in vitro screens for assessment of the drug activities for candidate compounds, evaluation of attractive candidate drugs with animal models, and most recently, a program to assist in translational research that leads to product development. Domestic and international sites also have clinical trial capabilities that can assist with studies, up through phase III trials. With this kind of assistance, the true cost of developing a drug is probably in the range of $15 million to $30 million (C. Nacy, Sequella Global Tuberculosis Foundation, unpublished data). To address the concern about the market for antituberculosis drugs, detailed studies are needed to characterize the markets outside of the established market economies. One estimate puts the global expenditure for the four main antituberculosis drugs at $800 million to $900 million per year, an amount that would definitely justify the development of new drugs in market terms.

Vaccine Development by Industry

To attempt to answer the question as to whether industry is actively pursuing development of candidate vaccines for tuberculosis prevention, the same 22 major pharmaceutical companies and 7 biotechnology companies that were mentioned above and that were questioned about new drug discovery were queried about any prospective vaccines. Twenty-one of the 22 companies contacted responded. There is clearly a paucity of activity in this area among established drug companies. Only two companies are involved in vaccine development. One is working on both a DNA-based vaccine and a vaccine with a live attenuated strain of the microorganism. In addition to a preventive vaccine, they are also exploring therapeutic use of their candidate vaccine in patients with established

M. tuberculosis infections. The second company is involved in vaccine development only in a very preliminary, exploratory fashion. It is working with a DNA-based vaccine that is in the public domain and is also interested in evaluating possible subunit vaccines.

Two of the seven biotechnology companies contacted indicated that their major activities are focused on the prevention or treatment of tuberculosis. For one company, the approach is exclusively vaccine development. It has developed a vaccine that uses three to five protective protein antigens made through the incorporation of the genes for these antigens (effectively, a synthetic gene) in one recombinant protein. The efficacy of this vaccine has been shown in a rodent model, and the safety of the vaccine has been demonstrated with monkeys. It expects clinical trials (phases I and II) to begin in about a year in several countries where the rate of endemic tuberculosis is high. The second biotechnology company is involved in the development of chemotherapeutic agents (ethambutol analogs and shikemic acid pathway inhibitors) as well as a candidate vaccine for the prevention of tuberculosis. This company is working with the experimental DNA vaccine described earlier (Lowrie et al., 1999).

In general, the time frame for full development, clinical testing, and final product marketing (if a successful vaccine were to be forthcoming) would be in the order of 10 to 20 years.

Private Foundations

Although the funding for research provided by private foundations is significantly less than that provided by government and industry, philanthropic foundations fill a crucial catalytic niche in many realms of medical research. Total philanthropic giving for 1997 came to $143.46 billion, with $121.89 billion from individuals and bequests, $13.37 billion from noncorporate foundations, and $8.2 billion from corporate foundations. Only 8.8 percent (just over $14 billion) of the total contributions received from charities was in the health category. These contributions included support for health services and health facilities, such as hospitals and nursing homes; support for organizations that address general health or specific diseases; and a small portion of support for medical research.

Grant-making organizations contributed $19.46 billion to nonprofit organizations in 1998, representing a 22 percent increase over 1977 contributions. Foundations currently spend 16.2 percent of total grant dollars, or $1.2 billion, on health. The majority of this (58 percent) goes to general and rehabilitative services, including hospitals and medical care, reproductive health, public health, health policy, and management. Only about $265 million, or 22 percent of the portion that foundations spent on health in 1998, went to medical research. In contrast, in 1998, government support for medical research was about $15 billion and industry support was $18 billion.

Although the amounts are relatively small, these funds provide crucial venture capital essential to the progress of medical research in many fields. In particular, private funders can move quickly to address new needs (particularly in translational research), take risks that potentially have high payoffs (for example, in behavioral research), and attempt novel funding approaches that may serve as a model for other funders.

Although comprehensive data that permit an examination of the categories of medical research that are funded are not available, an informal evaluation by the committee indicated that targeted support for tuberculosis is quite limited in light of the scope of the problem (Bond et al., 1998; Scott, 1999). The recent announcement by the Bill and Melinda Gates Foundation of grants for $50 million over 5 years for tuberculosis vaccine development may signal the start of interest in tuberculosis research by philanthropic foundations.

United States Agency for International Development

In light of the stated humanitarian and development goals of AID and its capacity to translate research advances into practice, its activities in tuberculosis have been extremely disappointing. Reducing the burden of disease would be of clear humanitarian benefit and would foster the sustained prosperity of nations with a high incidence of tuberculosis. However, AID has no tuberculosis program, and the past funding for tuberculosis that has been available has come through the HIV infection and AIDS program. One major AID activity has been the financial support of the global Stop TB Initiative. These funds have begun to build a framework for cooperation and collaboration among countries with a high incidence of tuberculosis, international organizations, and donors. A New Infectious Disease Initiative within AID has identified tuberculosis as one of its four components. However, a rational plan for the prioritization and implementation of these activities remains to be elucidated.

Food and Drug Administration

FDA has both intramural and extramural programs for tuberculosis research, although both are relatively small. The intramural program is centered within the Laboratory of Mycobacteria of the Center for Biologics Evaluation and Research. Funding for this program has steadily declined from about $235,000 in fiscal year 1995 to about $135,000 in fiscal year 2000. However, the program has been maintained through interagency agreements with NIH and the National Vaccine Program. The laboratory has worked on the generation of plasmids that carry key mycobacterial antigens, early development of vaccines that can be produced by edible plants, and evaluation of the protection conferred by auxotrophic live tuberculosis vaccines and DNA vaccines. Additional work has been conducted on virulence factors and mechanisms of protective immunity. This program, which is staffed by 10 individuals (FDA staff, fellows, and visiting scientists), has generated 24 publications over the last 3 years.

The extramural program is funded through the Orphan Drugs Program. Grants from this program are usually relatively small and are used to support early clinical work on new drugs. The program does not categorically fund tuberculosis research, and any application would be evaluated by external reviewers and ranked against all other applications. The program is not well known, and applications are not actively solicited.

RESEARCH PRIORITIES

In June 1985, CDC, NIH, the American Thoracic Society, and the Pittsfield Antituberculosis Association co-sponsored a conference to identify priority areas for research that might ultimately lead to the elimination of tuberculosis from the United States. This plan was incorporated into the ACET Strategic Plan for the Elimination of Tuberculosis in the United States (Centers for Disease Control, 1989) and was further elaborated in the Action Plan to Combat Multidrug-Resistant Tuberculosis (Centers for Disease Control and Prevention, 1992) The plan included an extensive list of investigative directions that should be pursued and a plea for their financial support. Reflecting on this list 15 years later is both discouraging and encouraging. It is discouraging to realize that virtually no funding and consequently no research was conducted for 7 years after its publication. It is encouraging to see that, following the expansion of funding that occurred between 1992 and 1995, there has been an explosion of knowledge and the development of a cohort of investigators and facilities in virtually every field of research relevant to tuberculosis control. Yet, the committee concludes that the level of support remains woefully inadequate, considering the global burden of disease and the potential of the current research network to make discoveries that will change the way the prevention, diagnosis, and treatment of tuberculosis are thought of.

The cost for the research plan in the Action Plan to Combat Multidrug-Resistant Tuberculosis was placed at about $160 million per year in 1984. At best the federal funding for research has been about half that amount. Since the development of the action plan, a *Blueprint for Tuberculosis Vaccine Development* was published 1998. That blueprint proposed a 20-year

$800 million budget, or about $40 million per year, for vaccine development. The estimate, however, seems to be based on the amount spent annually on the treatment of tuberculosis rather than on an objective costing of the plan. As discussed earlier, the committee recommends a similar initiative for the development of tests for the diagnosis of latent infection that would identify with a high sensitivity and high specificity, those who will develop tuberculosis and another initiative for the development of treatments for those with latent infections (i.e., drugs and immune modulators). That would yield a total budget of about $280 million per year for research to support the original items in the action plan: the vaccine initiative, the diagnostic test initiative, and the treatment initiative. This is the best estimate that the committee can make given the available information. Accurate budget estimates will be needed for all three initiatives to effectively argue for the funding of these programs.

In addition to obtaining appropriate amounts of funding, there are important issues related to the efficient use of those funds. The differences between the different funders and researchers involved in tuberculosis research provide both challenges and opportunities. It will be a challenge to ensure coordination and communication links along the entire pipeline from basic to operational research to maximize efficiency and minimize delays. These differences, however, also provide an unprecedented opportunity to achieve the goals outlined by this committee and prior bodies. Impediments must be replaced with incentives at each step in the process of the development of diagnostic tests, drugs, and vaccines.

Although the committee endorses the scope of the research agenda outlined in the *Strategic Plan for the Elimination of Tuberculosis* (Centers for Disease Control, 1989) and the clear prioritization relevant to vaccine production delineated in the *Blueprint for Tuberculosis Vaccine Development* (National Institutes of Health, 1998) (that vaccine development remains an important global priority), the single highest research priority is research relevant to the identification and treatment of tuberculosis infection. This focus is justified in light of the central importance of the diagnosis and treatment of tuberculosis infection to the elimination of tuberculosis from the United States. Although existing evidence and tools justify the expansion of targeted screening and treatment of latent tuberculosis infections now, better tools for the diagnosis of infection and drugs for the treatment of infected individuals would facilitate these activities. The diagnostic test might be approached as a two-step test, with the first step very sensitive and the second step highly specific. An action plan that delineates the short- and long-term strategies for achieving these goals, needs to be fully elucidated by the research community. It is anticipated that this strategy will include the following elements:

• The strategy will include NIH because the benefits of basic research cannot be anticipated and are difficult to predict and, thus, it is difficult to make specific recommendations. Nevertheless, the goal of eliminating tuberculosis infection from the United States must be made clear to independent investigators. The best way to ensure that the best minds of the current generation are focused on this goal is to make a sustained commitment to a staged, coordinated tripling of financial support for basic tuberculosis research that is likely to foster this goal. Realms to be supported by these funds must include definition of the bacteriology of "latent" infection and the identification of the pharmacological agents that kill latent bacilli. Specific immunological markers of infection need to be identified and immunological predictors of those individuals with latent tuberculosis who will later have active disease must be found. Funding for mathematical models that can be used to compare various interventions should be encouraged.

• Seed grant support for translating basic scientific knowledge into promising tests and compounds must be made available from governmental groups (e.g., through agencies of the Department of Health and Human Services, funding mechanisms such as Small Business Grants, and the Defense Advanced Research Projects Agency). The specifics of the potential market for a novel diagnostic test that can determine who among the millions of Americans at high risk of infection and an effective drug for the treatment of the millions who actually harbor *M. tuberculosis* must be emphasized to those who set industrial research priorities. Awareness of this market should drive small biotechnology companies into diagnostic assay development and the identification of new agents. The opportunity to test these diagnostic assays and drugs in cooperation with publicly funded networks of clinical trials should entice pharmaceutical and biotechnology companies to expand on the knowledge gained by publicly funded basic investigators and rapidly move new products through commercial development. Formation of a joint venture between industry and public sector agencies, would speed the attainment of this goal. Finally, a detailed study of the global market for licensed tuberculosis pharmaceutical and diagnostic products, along with information on the requirements for entering the largest markets could dispel the conventional wisdom that there is no market for tuberculosis drugs.

• A critical reappraisal of the CDC research agenda should be conducted. Its efforts should also be focused on its unique capacity to conduct pragmatic research linking expertise in study design with broad access to patients and clinical specimens to determine the performance characteristics of new laboratory technologies and the efficacies of new drugs. A diagnostics network, akin to the existing Tuberculosis Trials

Consortium, should be developed for the rapid assessment of new tools for the diagnosis of infection and disease. The Tuberculosis Trials Consortium, capable of enrolling large numbers of people each year, should be maintained and expanded to fill the gap between industry-driven product development and product implementation. In the short term, these efforts should be focused on evaluations of currently available agents, such as the use of fluoroquinolones and rifapentine, for treatment of infection. In addition to providing important information, these efforts will prime the pump for new agents as they become available, perhaps oxazolidinones. Intensive monitoring for adverse outcomes as they arise under operational conditions must be pursued before expansion of these programs. Subsequently, this network can be used to provide clinical confirmation of basic insights and advances. This network must reach out to community-based health care providers and for-profit health care providers.

• These clinical trials should be extended by AID to include sites in other countries with high rates of tuberculosis infection. These efforts not only would provide important information of relevance to the United States but would also demonstrate the potential of these technologies to improve the health of people in other countries, particularly those that account for considerable proportions of U.S. immigrants.

• Operational research must define efficient and cost-effective approaches to the implementation of these approaches, particularly in privatized health care delivery settings and medically marginalized populations.

Another area for increased attention is research related to the epidemiology of tuberculosis as the incidence declines and the disease approaches elimination. The focus of this research should be on distinguishing reactivation of latent infection from more recent transmission and will likely include more widespread genotyping and more traditional types of epidemiological studies. The results of that research should also then be translated into information that will be useful in guiding expanded contact investigations and the identification of outbreak situations.

Elimination of tuberculosis infection is an ambitious goal, but it is central to the elimination of tuberculosis. A sustained commitment to this goal will have considerable incidental benefits.

REFERENCES

American Thoracic Society and Centers for Disease Control and Prevention. 2000. Targeted tuberculosis testing and treatment of latent infection. *Am J Respir Crit Care Med* 161:5221–5247.

Anonymous. 1997. Rapid diagnostic tests for tuberculosis. What is the appropriate use? *Am J Respir Crit Care Med* 155:1804–1814.

Aronson N, Santosham M, Howard R, Comstock G, and Harrison, L. 1999. The long-term efficacy of BCG vaccine. Abstracts of the 39th Interscience Conference on Antimicrobial Agents and Chemotherapy, September 1999. Washington, DC: American Society for Microbiology.

Behr MA, Warren SA, Salamon H, Hopewell PC, Ponce de Leon A, Daley CL, and Small PM. 1999. Transmission of *Mycobacterium tuberculosis* from patients smear-negative for acid-fast bacilli. *Lancet* 353:444–449.

Bond EC, Peck MG, and Scott, MB. 1998. The future of philanthropic support for research. *Scientist* 13(21):15.

Centers for Disease Control. 1989. A strategic plan for the elimination of tuberculosis in the United States. *MMWR* 38 (S3):1–25.

Centers for Disease Control and Prevention. 1992. National action plan to combat multidrug-resistant tuberculosis in the United States. *MMWR* 41(RR11):1–48.

Centers for Disease Control and Prevention. 1993. Recommendations of the International Task Force for Disease Eradication. *MMWR* 42(RR16):1–25.

Centers for Disease Control and Prevention. 1995. Improving tuberculosis treatment and control: An agenda behavioral, social, and health services research. Proceedings for "Tuberculosis and Behavior, National Workshop on Research for the 21st Century, 1995." Atlanta: Centers for Disease Control and Prevention.

Centers for Disease Control and Prevention. 1996. The role of BCG vaccine in the prevention and control of tuberculosis in the United States. *MMWR* 45 (RR4):1–18.

Centers for Disease Control and Prevention. 1998. Population-Based Survey for Drug Resistance of Tuberculosis—Mexico, 1997. *MMWR* 47:371–375.

Centers for Disease Control and Prevention. 2000. Targeted testing and treatment of latent tuberculosis infection. *MMWR* 49(RR-6):1–54.

Colditz GA, Brewer TF, Berkey CS, et al. 1994. Efficacy of BCG vaccine in the prevention of tuberculosis. Meta-analysis of the published literature. *JAMA* 271(9):698–702.

Crawford JT. 1994. New technologies in the diagnosis of tuberculosis. *Semin Respir Infect* 9:62(70.

Cynamon MH, Klemens SP, Sharpe CA, and Chase S. 1999. Activities of several novel oxazolidinones against *Mycobacterium tuberculosis* in a murine model. *Antimicrob Agents Chemother* 43:1189(1190.

Holden, M, Dubin MR, and Diamond PH. 1971. Frequency of negative intermediate-strength tuberculin sensitivity in persons with active tuberculosis. *N Engl J Med* 285:1506–1509.

Huebner RE, Schein MF, and Bass JB, Jr. 1993. The tuberculin skin test. *Clin Infect Dis* 17:968–975.

Iseman MD and Sbarbaro JA. 1991. Short-course chemotherapy of tuberculosis. Hail Britannia (and friends!). *Am Rev Respir Dis* 143(4):697–698.

Lowrie DB, Tascon RE, Bonato VL, et al. 1999. Therapy of tuberculosis in mice by DNA vaccination. *Nature* 400(6741):269–271.

National Institutes of Health. 1998. *Blueprint for Vaccine Development*. Report of a workshop held March 5–6, 1998, Rockville, MD.

NIAID. 2000. Blueprint of tuberculosis vaccine development. *Clinical Infectious Diseases* Vol. 30, Supp. 3 (June 2000), 5233–5242.

Nunn DR, and Douglas JE. 1980. Anergy in active pulmonary tuberculosis: A comparison between positive and negative reactors and evaluation of 5 TU and 250 TU skin test doses. *Chest* 77:32–37.

Pablos-Méndez A, Raviglione MC, Laszlo A, et al. 1998. Global surveillance for antituberculosis drug resistance, 1994–1997. World Health Organization-International Union Against Tuberculosis and Lung Disease. Working Group on Antituberculosis Drug Resistance Surveillance. *N Engl J Med* 338(23):164–169.

Raviglione M, Dye C, Schmidt S, and Kochi A. 1997. Assessment of worldwide tuberculosis control. *Lancet* 350:624–629.

Rodrigues LC, Diwan VK, and Wheeler JG. 1993. Protective effect of BCG against tuberculosis meningitis and miliary tuberculosis: A meta-analysis. *Int J Epidemiol* 22(6):1154–1158.

Scott, MB. 1999. *The Scientist* Oct 25:13.

Sterne JAC, Rodrigues LC, and Guedes IN. 1998. Does the efficacy of BCG decline with time since vaccination? *Int J Tuberc Lung Dis* 2:200–207.

Streeton JA, Desem N, and Jones SL. 1998. Sensitivity and specificity of a gamma interferon blood test for tuberculosis infection. *Int J Tuberc Lung Dis* 2:443–450.

6

The U.S. Role in Global
Tuberculosis Control

Tuberculosis is a leading cause of death worldwide, even though it is a readily treatable and preventable disease. Although an altruistic argument for promoting the global control of tuberculosis can easily be advanced, worldwide control of this disease is also in the nation's self-interest. The proportion of foreign-born tuberculosis patients in the United States has been steadily increasing. In 1998, 41 percent of all tuberculosis patients were foreign-born. It benefits the United States to help strengthen tuberculosis control programs globally, particularly in the countries that are the source of most tuberculosis cases imported into the United States. Tuberculosis will not be eliminated in the United States until the worldwide epidemic is brought under control. This chapter outlines the contributions that the United States can make to this effort.

RECOMMENDATIONS

Recommendation 6.1 To decrease the number of foreign-born individuals with tuberculosis in the United States, to minimize the spread and impact of multidrug-resistant tuberculosis, and to improve global health, the committee recommends that

• **The United States expand and strengthen its role in global tuberculosis control efforts, contributing to these efforts in a substantial manner through bilateral and multilateral international efforts.**

- **The United States contribute to global tuberculosis control efforts through targeted use of financial, technical, and human resources and research, all guided by a carefully considered strategic plan.**
- **The United States work in close coordination with other government and international agencies. In particular, the United States should continue its active role in and support of the Stop TB Initiative.**
- **The U.S. Agency for International Development (AID), the Centers for Disease Control and Prevention (CDC), and the National Institutes of Health (NIH) should jointly develop and publish strategic plans to guide U.S. involvement in global tuberculosis control efforts.**

GLOBAL CONTEXT OF TUBERCULOSIS

Even from the perspective of a developed country, such as the United States, it is increasingly clear that tuberculosis must be viewed in a global context to have a full understanding of the epidemiology of the disease and to develop effective strategies for its control. In the United States, as well as in other countries in which the incidence of tuberculosis is low (less than 25 cases per 100,000 population per year), increasing proportions of the new cases are occurring among individuals born in countries with a high incidence of tuberculosis. Although it is frequently stated that tuberculosis has undergone a resurgence in industrialized countries, at least in part it would be more accurate to view the increases that occurred in the late 1980s and early 1990s as a consequence of shifting global patterns of the disease. No longer are populations and the diseases prevalent within them forced by circumstances to remain in the countries or areas where they originate. Diseases such as tuberculosis are not constrained by national boundaries any more than people are constrained by national boundaries. Thus, in addition to the factors that influence rates of disease in a given country, the global distribution of tuberculosis is also influenced by the factors that determine the movements of populations in general. This is true for at least two reasons. First, in many areas of the world the majority of adults, not just a small subgroup, have latent tuberculosis infection. Second, tuberculosis infection causes no symptoms and results in no alteration in activities; consequently, movement is not limited.

A number of the factors that have been identified as predispositions to the emergence of "new" pathogens have also influenced the spread of tuberculosis (Stephens et al., 1998). Population movements within and between countries both shift persons from high- to low-incidence countries and cause increased crowding in urban areas, thereby facilitating tuberculosis transmission. Increasing economic gradients increase the allure of wealthier countries for poor people in the developing world. In many parts of the world, wars, worsening economic circumstances, reordering of priorities, and lack of political commitment have all led to deterioration in the public health infrastructure while, at the same time, the need for disease control programs and surveillance is increasing. Consequently, overall, there are probably more cases of tuberculosis in the world today than there have ever been. It would be easy to blame human immunodeficiency virus (HIV) infection for the world's worsening tuberculosis situation, and, clearly, it is an important factor. However, one could contend that HIV merely illuminated the existing weaknesses of existing tuberculosis control programs.

In view of the current state of global tuberculosis control efforts, it is not surprising that in low-incidence countries, increasing proportions of new cases are arising from among individuals born in high-incidence areas. In general, low-incidence, industrialized countries have in place screening processes by which applicants for immigrant visas are examined for tuberculosis and individuals with infectious tuberculosis are denied visas. However, the systems are imperfect and, depending on the circumstances, may break down entirely. For example, because of the need for rapid resettlement of a large number of Southeast Asian refugees in the United States in the late 1970s, screening for tuberculosis was not performed. As a consequence, persons with active tuberculosis entered the country, resulting in a reduction of the previous years' rate of decline and an actual slight increase in the number of cases of tuberculosis in 1980. San Francisco was the destination for many of the refugees, and the number of cases rose from approximately 300 in 1978 to 400 in 1979 to 500 in 1980. A similar impact on case numbers was seen in Hawaii with the unannounced arrival of a large number of Filipino World War II veterans who much earlier had been promised citizenship in return for serving in the U.S. armed forces.

The combination of the natural history of tuberculosis, with its often long period of latency and the high prevalence of both latent infection and disease in many parts of the world, together with the many factors that cause individuals and groups of people to move from country to country ideally suits global distribution of the disease. The phenomenon of the globalization of tuberculosis is clearly seen in most industrialized countries. In the United States foreign-born persons made up 41 percent of the new cases reported in 1998 (see Chapter 2). During the 1990s, this proportion has progressively increased, in part because the intensified control measures applied early in the 1990s were directed more toward U.S.-born individuals. As noted in Chapter 2, the proportion of cases among U.S.-

born persons decreased by 44 percent between 1992 and 1998, whereas there was a 4 percent increase in the proportion among the foreign-born population (Centers for Disease Control and Prevention, 1999). A similar impact has been described in other industrialized countries (Raviglione, 1993).

The conclusion is inescapable that globalization is inevitable, and unless the United States is going to close its borders, the control and ultimate elimination of tuberculosis in the United States will require vast improvements in global tuberculosis control efforts. At this point the outlook is not good for any substantial improvements in tuberculosis control in high-incidence countries unless there is considerable new external assistance.

GLOBAL TUBERCULOSIS CONTROL EFFORTS

To meet the challenge of tuberculosis there must be developed within the world community a sense of shared responsibility and mutual confidence to mount a global tuberculosis control program. A commitment to basic, translational (from research laboratory to clinical practice), and operational research is essential. In addition to research there must be a commitment to training. A trained cadre of clinicians and scientists is essential for implementation of control measures, evaluation of their effectiveness, and development of new knowledge (see Chapter 3).

The global epidemic of tuberculosis presents a dynamic and evolving situation. It must be met with a new level of international commitment and collaboration, with assiduous application of existing tools and with new knowledge and approaches. Tuberculosis is not like smallpox, which was eradicated by a massive but short-term campaign. Tuberculosis control requires patience, persistence, and continued emphasis on the provision of more permanent systems of care. This can be accomplished only by a coordinated global approach with effective partnership between developing and industrialized countries (see the box Pedro's and Juan's Stories).

Given this context and overall framework, what is the role of the United States in global tuberculosis control? In general terms the United States should have concerns founded in self-interest and humanitarianism. These concerns, however, are not the polar opposites that they might seem. The unity of self-interest and humanitarianism is perhaps best conveyed by a quote from an earlier Institute of Medicine (IOM) report, *The Future of Public Health*, (Institute of Medicine, 1988) "The direct interests of the American people are best served when the U.S. acts decisively to promote health around the world." Furthermore, it is stated in the same publication, "The failure to engage in the fight to anticipate, prevent, and advocate global health problems would diminish America's stature in the realm of health, and jeopardize our own health, economy and national security."

Despite the very strong arguments that can be mounted for the justification of foreign assistance, the United States contributes a smaller percentage (0.1 percent) of its gross national product to overseas aid than any of the other countries in the Organization for Economic Cooperation and Development. Moreover, of the total of $9.9 billion for foreign assistance provided by the United States in 1994, only $1 billion was for health-related activities.

The IOM report cited above presents a compelling, eloquent, and well-documented case for the involvement of the United States in global health as a general concern. Such involvement, the report argues, serves to protect the U.S. population, enhance the U.S. economy, and advance the international interests of the United States. Virtually all of the generic arguments could also be made specifically for tuberculosis but will not be repeated here. However, it has only been in the past few years that governmental agencies, as well as nongovernmental organizations (NGOs), in the United States have taken any interest in tuberculosis beyond our borders. Currently, and for the past several years, funds that are specifically targeted for international tuberculosis activities have been appropriated to AID and CDC, although the amounts are quite small.

It is possible to argue that, on grounds of narrow self-interest, the United States and other industrialized nations should be concerned with tuberculosis abroad because it is not possible to erect a protective cordon sanitaire. This is especially the case with tuberculosis at the border, as is the case with the United States and Mexico. To so frame the issue, however, is to unduly restrict the moral vision of the United States. Eight million cases of tuberculosis annually and 2 million to 3 million deaths a year demand U.S. attention, regardless of their ultimate impact on the well-being of Americans. The United States shares with other industrialized nations the obligation to shoulder the task of fostering the development of new drugs and therapies for the treatment of tuberculosis, new tools for the diagnosis of tuberculosis, and an antituberculosis vaccine. Only the industrialized nations have the scientific, technological, and financial resources necessary to make possible the long-term effort that vaccine development will require. It is that capacity that imposes on the United States the moral duty to act to save the lives of millions who would otherwise die. That the national epidemiological interests are also well served by intelligent efforts to contain tuberculosis adds to the compelling case for U.S. involvement.

NIH has also recently begun to support tuberculosis research projects that are based in developing countries and that target research questions

Pedro's and Juan's Stories

One of the most important roles of the CURE-TB Binational Referral System is educating tuberculosis patients about their disease and the importance of finishing the prescribed treatment. Pedro's and Lupe's stories are examples of how CURE-TB helps patients finish their treatment.

Pedro

Pedro was diagnosed with tuberculosis in April 1998 in a northern California county. He was started on medications and left for Jalisco, Mexico, a week later. The California doctor sent a referral to CURE-TB, and CURE-TB staff contacted Pedro in Jalisco via telephone. At the same time, CURE-TB notified the Mexican National Tuberculosis Program of Pedro's arrival in Jalisco.

Pedro informed CURE-TB staff that upon his arrival he had visited a local clinic, where he was evaluated by available diagnostic procedures (sputum smear tests and a clinical evaluation) and was told that he did not appear to have tuberculosis. CURE-TB staff asked Pedro for the local clinic's number to provide his Mexican physician with Pedro's past medical history. CURE-TB counselors immediately called Pedro's physician to provide information on Pedro's previous diagnostic studies, which included culture results positive for *Mycobacterium tuberculosis*, and his treatment course while he was in the United States. Pedro's physician appreciated this information and decided to continue Pedro's treatment. CURE-TB staff communicated with Pedro again to let him know that he needed to visit his physician as soon as possible.

A month later, CURE-TB staff received the final results on Pedro's tuberculosis drug resistance tests from the California clinic. Pedro's infecting *M. tuberculosis* strain was resistant to one drug, isoniazid. This was immediately communicated to Pedro's physician, who added ethambutol to his original three-drug regimen. Pedro finished his treatment in November 1998 and is one of the success stories of the CURE-TB referral system. The county in California where Pedro currently resides

---

relevant to areas with a high incidence of tuberculosis. The greatest strength of the U.S. vis-à-vis other countries is its scientific and technological capacity. The United States should take a lead role in basic investigation of tuberculosis. NIH should be the lead agency in this undertaking but should work in close collaboration with the Research and Development Unit of the World Health Organization (WHO) in defining a coordinated global research strategy. The focus of this basic research effort should be on the development of new tools that can be used against tuberculosis. These include new diagnostic tests, new drugs, and an effective vaccine. Development efforts in these areas, in addition to requiring strong efforts in the basic sciences, will also entail participation by private industry. To foster these specific research endeavors a coordinating council that would include NIH, CDC, WHO, industry, and NGOs should be

after returning from Jalisco was also informed of his successful completion of the treatment.

Juan

In May 1999, the Los Angeles County tuberculosis Program informed the CURE-TB system about a symptomatic contact of one of their patients, Lupe. The contact, Lupe's brother, Juan, was living in Michoacan, Mexico. Lupe reported that she had lived with Juan months earlier, before she traveled to the United States, and that he had been sick and coughing at that time.

CURE-TB notified national and state health officials in Mexico about Juan's suspect status. CURE-TB also contacted Juan directly by phone and he informed them that he was indeed ill but that he was moving to the United States within the week. Juan was provided with information about the available tuberculosis services at his intended U.S. destination and was urged to seek care immediately upon his arrival. Within days of his arrival Juan did indeed visit a health center and was found to have infectious tuberculosis. He was started on treatment and directly observed treatment regimen.

In this case CURE-TB was able to facilitate rapid access to appropriate care for a symptomatic individual. Not only was the patient able to get the care he needed, but a potential source of prolonged transmission in the community was averted. In addition, Mexican health authorities were able to conduct a contact investigation in Michoacan. Both countries and families on both sides of the United States-Mexico border were able to benefit from the interventions of the CURE-TB system.

Cases such as Juan's and Pedro's are common to the CURE-TB system. The exchange of information between providers, as well as patient education and guidance, are essential factors for the successful completion of treatment for tuberculosis patients moving between the United States and Mexico. CURE-TB staff are committed and eager to continue providing these services.

developed. This group should develop a specific tuberculosis research agenda and a strategic plan for achieving it, including advocacy efforts to generate funding.

The research agenda should include not only basic research but also the capacity to undertake applied investigations including clinical trials. In this area of investigation the U.S.-based organization should coordinate both with WHO and with NGOs that are in a position to facilitate and participate in such studies. A major component of applied research should be research training and building of research capacity in developing countries.

In addition to providing leadership in the science of tuberculosis, the United States should do several other things. First, it should take the lead in developing incentives for research and development within private industry and for developing pricing schemes that would allow innovations to be affordable in high-incidence countries. Such incentives should build upon those already in the Orphan Drug Act and could take the form of, for example, an extension of patent rights on any new products or the implementation of mechanisms to ensure the protection of intellectual property rights. With regard to affordability, tiered pricing schemes could be developed and supported internationally. Additional mechanisms that should be explored include the development of a large central purchase pool fund for drugs and diagnostic tools with a guaranteed volume of sales.

Training and education is a second area of major importance in which the United States should be involved. As with research, the United States should work in close coordination with WHO and NGOs involved in tuberculosis training in developing countries, especially the International Union Against Tuberculosis and Lung Disease and the Royal Netherlands Antituberculosis Association. With regard to education and training, U.S.-based education must overcome a significant barrier. In many quarters it is believed that the United States has little to offer to people from high-incidence countries because different approaches to education are used in the United States. Only by progressive involvement in training efforts will this attitude be overcome. The particular area of strength of U.S.-based or U.S.-conducted training is in the area of research. Currently, Fogarty International Center of NIH, with funding from AID, is supporting the training of investigators. Such training should be maintained, if not expanded, and should target persons from high-incidence countries.

A planning process should define the roles and responsibilities of various organizations involved in the training of individuals involved in tuberculosis control. This process would include the organizations mentioned above as well as people from high-incidence countries. These international training plans should take into account of and should be incorporated into the strategic training plans (for providers, patients, and the public) mentioned in Chapter 3.

A third area in which the United States should play a prominent role in global tuberculosis control is leadership. As noted above the United States is not perceived as having much to offer other than financial resources and basic research. This, however, is clearly not the case. United States-based agencies and organizations are viewed as world leaders in many areas. From this position these same agencies and organizations can operate to mobilize similar agencies and organizations globally in support of tuberculosis control activities. To gain the trust of the tuberculosis control community, however, it is essential that United States-based agencies and organizations operate within a coordinated overall framework. Such a framework is in the process of being developed. The Stop TB Initiative is a partnership hosted by WHO that seeks to accelerate global tuberculosis control via a coordinated multisectoral effort. Funding provided by AID served to catalyze the development of the initiative.

The willingness of the United States to support the use of both patient-centered therapy and fixed-dose medications is vital to their adoption by countries experiencing high rates of tuberculosis, thereby strengthening efforts to eliminate tuberculosis within the borders of the United States. Immigrants, refugees, tourists, and students bring with them both their country's rates of tuberculosis and rates of drug resistance.

Ideally, all tuberculosis patients would be enrolled in well-organized and adequately funded programs. However, there will be occasions and circumstances in which directly observed therapy is not a viable option. The establishment of fixed-dose combination medications as the only acceptable standard of care when directly observed therapy is not available could benefit tuberculosis control both in the United States and throughout the world. Encouraging the removal of rifampin and other single-drug antituberculosis medications from the open markets of countries with a high incidence of tuberculosis and from direct access of physicians who are not trained as tuberculosis specialists could further enhance this tuberculosis control effort.

The United States can also assert leadership by the strategic use of technical and financial assistance. AID is critical in this regard. Only recently has AID begun to exploit its presence in high-incidence countries to address tuberculosis. Ongoing efforts are limited to India, El Salvador, Mexico, Kazakhstan, Russia, and South Africa. The largest effort to date has been the development of a center in Tamil Nadu, India, that is focused on the implementation and evaluation of a model DOTS program. A New Infectious Disease Initiative has identified tuberculosis as one of its four components. However, a rational plan for prioritizing and implementing these activites remains to be elucidated, and at this point, there is little central coordination of funding of tuberculosis control projects by AID, thus precluding a strategic approach. The agency should develop more effective mechanisms for internal coordination and develop its own strategic plan that will enable its assistance to be used most effectively.

United States-based foundations could also be used in a strategic manner to fund tuberculosis control programs or elements of programs in high-incidence countries. Given the wealth and power of some foundations, their involvement could have substantial impacts. The Stop TB Initiative that would target foundations with specific requests upon which there is a strong global consensus should develop a funding plan.

To again quote the IOM report on *The Future of Public Health*, "Our nation's vital interests are clearly best served by sustained and strengthened U.S. engagement in global health" (Institute of Medicine, 1998). There is no better example of a situation to which the statement applies than global tuberculosis control.

REFERENCES

Centers for Disease Control and Prevention. 1999. *Reported Tuberculosis.* Atlanta: Centers for Disease Control and Prevention.

Institute of Medicine. 1988. *The Future of Public Health.* Washington, DC: National Academy Press.

Raviglione MC, Sudre P, Rieder HL, Spinaci S, and Kochi A. 1993. Secular trends of tuberculosis in western Europe. *Bull WHO* 71(3–4):297–306.

Stephens DS, Moxon ER, Adams J, et al. 1998. Emerging and reemerging infectious diseases: A multidisciplinary perspective. *Am J Med Sci* 315(2):64–75.

7

Mobilizing for Elimination

The United States has a long history of social mobilization efforts in support of tuberculosis control. Social mobilization provides for the enlistment and coordination of efforts by myriad groups and individuals. Advocacy to influence policy makers and education of patients, health care providers, and the general public are critical activities. A World Health Organization ad hoc committee identified the lack of political will on the part of national governments as a fundamental constraint to developing and sustaining effective tuberculosis control programs. Social mobilization is necessary to build and sustain political will in the United States and can lead similar efforts internationally. This chapter reviews social mobilization efforts related to tuberculosis in the United States and outlines strategies that can be used to support a tuberculosis elimination effort.

RECOMMENDATIONS

Recommendation 7.1 To build public support and sustain public interest and commitment to the elimination of tuberculosis, the committee recommends that the Centers for Disease Control and Prevention (CDC) significantly increase resources for activities to secure and sustain public understanding and support for tuberculosis elimination efforts at the national, state, and local levels, including programs to increase knowledge among targeted groups of the general public.

Recommendation 7.2 To increase the effectiveness of mobilization efforts the committee recommends that the National Coalition for the Elimination of Tuberculosis continue to provide leadership and oversight and that CDC continue to work in collaboration with the coalition to secure the support and participation of nontraditional public health partners, ensure the development of state and local coalitions, and evaluate public understanding and support for tuberculosis elimination efforts, with the assistance of public opinion research experts.

Recommendation 7.3 To assess the impacts of these recommendations and to measure progress toward accomplishing the elimination of tuberculosis, the committee recommends that, 3 years after the publication of this report and periodically thereafter, the Office of the Secretary of Health and Human Services conduct an evaluation of the actions taken in response to the recommendations in this report.

Social mobilization has been identified as a vital prerequisite to accelerating the decline of tuberculosis in the United States. In March 1998, the World Health Organization convened an ad hoc committee on tuberculosis to analyze individual countries' abilities to reach year 2000 targets for tuberculosis control. Although the committee's focus was on the 22 so-called high burden countries that account for the majority of the world's burden of tuberculosis, the committee's major findings also apply to low-burden countries such as the United States. The committee found:

> Intensified technical efforts will not by themselves bring about the acceleration and expansion needed for tuberculosis control programs. This Committee has identified six principal constraints regarding action by health authorities. These are financial shortages, human resource problems, organizational factors, lack of a secure supply of quality anti-TB drugs, and public information gaps about TB's danger. *The most fundamental constraint is the lack of political will to develop and sustain effective TB programs.* (Emphasis added) (World Health Organization, 1998)

The Ad Hoc Committee identified four factors important to creating and sustaining political will:

1. Popular Perception: The public should recognize tuberculosis as a priority problem with an achievable solution.
2. Technical Consensus. The consensus among the technical and scientific communities is thought to be indispensable. Such consensus al-

lows for consistent information to reach policy makers across all levels of government

3. External Concern. External concern relies on the use of community leaders to communicate need to policy makers.

4. Media Interest. The Committee found the use of the media to create a climate of public interest and concern critical to sustaining policy maker and government interest.

All four factors represent challenges in social mobilization in the United States. Public opinion research clearly shows that the popular perception of tuberculosis is that it is not a problem in the United States (CDC, unpublished data). In part this is due to the demographics of the disease, the majority of those afflicted with tuberculosis are at the margins of society, and to the fact that the disease is once again in decline. There is a technical consensus around tuberculosis as represented by the guidelines jointly endorsed by the American Thoracic Society, the Centers for Disease Control and Prevention, the American Academy of Pediatrics, and the Infectious Diseases Society. However, there has been difficulty communicating this consensus while maintaining media interest. News coverage naturally gravitates to unusual and exciting situations. For example, although there is technical consensus that the risk for tuberculosis infection aboard airplanes is low, news coverage has made some people afraid to fly. In another example, although multidrug resistant tuberculosis is a very serious problem, with a potential to worsen in the future, it represents a small and decreasing number of cases in the United States. Still the news media devotes a large part of its coverage to this type of tuberculosis, which generates a frenzied call for tuberculin skin testing in suburban schools. Media interest has to be maintained while communicating information accurately. Finally, external concern is very weak at the national level. Since the American Tuberculosis Association became the American Lung Association, the Christmas Seal Campaign and the selection of the national chairman has focused on other issues other than tuberculosis. External concern has generally tended to come from local groupings and ad hoc alliances. The funding increase for tuberculosis in the 1990s is in large part attributable to the interaction between tuberculosis and HIV. Because of this interaction, AIDS activists provided support for the TB community in obtaining more resources. On a local level, a number of state and city lung associations are active advocates and supporters of the tuberculosis program. In South Carolina, the Lung Association has provided resources for the incentives and enablers program that has served as a model to much of the rest of the nation. In California, as described in the site visit notes, the San Diego Lung Association has been a key supporter in the housing program and in developing community

The Impact of Social Mobilization

In 1944, the U.S. Congress passed the Public Health Service Act, which in part, authorized the establishment of a federal Tuberculosis Control Program. The program provided grants to state health departments for tuberculosis control activities. In 1961, Congress approved legislation providing additional funds through categorical grants. At the height of the "project grant" era in 1969, the annual rate of reduction of new cases was 8.2 percent.

The Program was phased out with no monies available after 1972. By 1980, the impact of the phase-out was apparent—the annual rate of reduction of new cases had slowed to 5.1 percent and new cases actually increased 2% for African Americans.

The American Lung Association (ALA) made the re-creation of a separate funding authority for tuberculosis a priority throughout the 1970s. The momentum of the program was lost, however, and the rate reduction slowed even further and by 1982 was only 3.2 percent.

ALA increased its social mobilization and advocacy efforts in late 1980 with the opening of a full-time office in Washington, D.C. It first priority was tuberculosis funding. In April 1981 ALA sponsored its first Advocacy Leadership Conference for its state and local associations. Plans were made to approach the tuberculosis funding issue using all available legislative vehicles.

Representative Henry Waxman of California, Chair of the House Subcommittee on Health, sponsored legislation to authorize Tuberculosis Project Grants, and ALA's nationwide volunteer core was mobilized. Unfortunately, the 96th U.S. Congress failed to act.

At the beginning of the 97th U.S. Congress Mr. Waxman again introduced legislation. But this time, ALA volunteers in Utah secured an agreement from Senator Orrin Hatch (Chair of the Senate Committee on Labor and Human Resources) to sponsor similar legislation in the Senate. ALA also mobilized other organizations, including the American Public Health Association as well as the ALA's own medical section, the American Thoracic Society. The media was enlisted to educate the public and policy makers about the problem of tuberculosis in key communities as well as nationwide. Much of the mobilization effort centered on explaining the problems of tuberculosis in refugee populations.

support for the tuberculosis program. Finally, a recently formed coalition in Washington State has been an effective advocate for the tuberculosis program.

To sustain adequate political will, social mobilization becomes a critical component in any effort to eliminate tuberculosis (see the box The Impact of Social Mobilization). The purpose of such mobilization is to help build and sustain adequate political and financial support by key leaders and policy makers as well as to engage the active participation and cooperation of health care providers, members of high-risk groups, and patients themselves in a combined assault on the disease.

In August 1981, 250 congressional conferees agreed to the conference report for H.R. 3982 just prior to the summer recess. The Program for Tuberculosis Project Grants was authorized at $9 million in fiscal year 1982, $10 million in fiscal year 1983, and $11 million in fiscal year 1984. However, no funds were included in any of the appropriations bills going forward.

In March 1982, at a conference marking the 100th anniversary of the date that Robert Koch presented his now famous paper on the etiology of tuberculosis, ALA launched plans to secure an appropriation for the new program. A presidential veto of the final fiscal year 1982 Supplemental Appropriations bill allowed ALA to mobilize one last time. The effort succeeded with the signing, in September 1982, of the final fiscal year 1982 Supplemental Appropriations bill which provided $1 million for tuberculosis control efforts. Following shortly thereafter was an appropriation for fiscal year 1983 of $5 million.

ALA's mobilization campaign resulted in a clear awareness by Congress of the tuberculosis problem and the national commitment needed for its control. The House Report for the fiscal year 1982 Supplemental Appropriations bill noted:

> The additional funds are to be used for tuberculosis control activities. The Committee is concerned about the incidence of Tuberculosis in this country. Over the past three year, there has been a leveling off of the slow but steady decline in tuberculosis cases which had been evident in the country for decades. The disease continues to be a major health problem despite the fact that medical research has provided us with effective methods for its prevention and control. Our failure to prevent and control Tuberculosis is measure by the 27,412 new cases reported in 1981.

The Senate Report for the FY 82 Supplemental bill noted:

> Each year nearly 30,000 people develop tuberculosis and require long-term treatment. For nearly three decades the number of cases in the United States has been decreasing, but this trend has stopped and essentially leveled off since 1979. Also, of concern to the Committee is that people living in our cities are at nearly twice the risk of the general population. The problem is further complicated by drug resistance, new sources of infection, and most disturbing, the transmission of the disease to children.

Mobilization involves the enlistment and coordination of efforts by myriad groups and persons, including nontraditional partners outside of the public and private health sectors. It includes advocacy to influence policy makers as well as education of patients, high-risk groups, health care providers and the general public. To build the level of political will that is required, all relevant sectors of society are needed to help and must be convinced that it is in their interest to achieve this worthwhile goal.

The United States has a long history of social mobilization efforts tied to tuberculosis control. The National Association for the Study and Prevention of Tuberculosis (NASPT) used social mobilization techniques to promote the establishment of public health departments and tuberculosis control programs in every community in the country at the beginning of the 20th century. The NASPT also urged the use of taxes to make tuberculosis care free to all patients.

An important undertaking of NASPT was surveys documenting the morbidity and mortality from tuberculosis (see Chapter 2). These surveys served many purposes. First, they provided much needed information to the public about tuberculosis and the difficulties that its control presented. More important, however, the surveys formed the basis for the first social mobilization efforts, sponsored by NASPT, to increase public funding for tuberculosis control.

In 1916, NASPT passed a resolution calling for federal government participation in tuberculosis control, indicating that it is "desirable and necessary" and that "the proper federal agency for the purpose is the U.S. Public Health Service" (Shyrock, 1957). That year, a bill providing that a division of tuberculosis control be set up in the U.S. Public Health Service was introduced in the U.S. House of Representatives. It was not until 1944, however, that such a division was created. Federal funding of state tuberculosis efforts began in 1961. However, after a decade of support, funding was phased out when all state categorical public health funding was consolidated into block grants.

Organizations sponsoring the majority of the early social mobilization efforts turned to other public health priorities, and policy makers grew complacent as a result of the steady 5–6% annual decline in case rates. By the late 1970s, little federal or state funding was dedicated to tuberculosis control (see Chapter 2).

In 1982, the U.S. Congress authorized once again a dedicated source of funding for tuberculosis control programs, Project Grants for Tuberculosis Preventive Health Projects (Public Health Service Act 42 section 317 E). Without the social mobilization efforts and political will of earlier in the century, funding for fiscal year 1982 was set at $1 million. The continued lack of social mobilization efforts would result in the continued low level of funding as the resurgence of tuberculosis appeared.

In 1984, James Mason, who was then director of the Centers for Disease Control, called upon the public health community to develop a plan for the elimination of tuberculosis in the United States. The resulting report *A Strategic Plan for the Elimination of Tuberculosis in the United States* (Centers for Disease Control, 1989), was published in April 1989. The plan provided a detailed road map for the re-creation of the public health infrastructure critical to the control of tuberculosis. More importantly, the plan recognized the integral relationship between appropriate social mobilization and the sustainability of political will key to effective tuberculosis control (Centers for Disease Control, 1989).

Although identified as a methodology for technology assessment and transfer, the voluntary sector was challenged to revitalize social mobilization efforts, including education and advocacy activities. This sector was also called upon to form coalitions in support of increased resources for tuberculosis control programs. The media was also called upon to provide appropriate coverage on the advances in the diagnosis, treatment, and prevention of tuberculosis to increase support for tuberculosis programs (Centers for Disease Control, 1989).

The National Coalition for the Elimination of Tuberculosis (NCET) was established by the American Lung Association with support from the Robert Wood Johnson Foundation to reengineer the social mobilization effort. The mobilization efforts of NCET combined with the blueprint for program design in the strategic plan are, in large part, responsible for the significant increase in tuberculosis control resources described in Chapter 2 (see the box National Coalition to Eliminate Tuberculosis).

The need for social mobilization is again recognized in the revision of the strategic plan, *Tuberculosis Elimination Revisited: Obstacles, Opportunities and a Renewed Commitment* (Centers for Disease Control, 1999). NCET is challenged to continue to advocate for resources for effective tuberculosis control and is called upon to expand partnerships not only at the state and local levels, but also with nontraditional partners (Centers for Disease Control, 1999).

To reinvigorate social mobilization efforts for tuberculosis control, specific strategies must be devised for reaching each of the groups in the public and private sectors. The national goal for eliminating tuberculosis and its rationale must be articulated clearly and publicized widely so that the goal is understood and sufficiently supported. Progress toward achieving the goal must also be communicated to these groups. A set of no more than three or four simple indicators of progress toward tuberculosis elimination (as described in Chapter 3) should be developed and widely published so that progress or its absence are clear to all. Also, a review of progress toward accomplishing the goals set forth in this report, conducted through the Office of the Secretary of Health and Human Services, should be conducted 3 years from the publication of this report. Again, the progress or lack thereof should be widely published. Specific target audiences and objectives for mobilization include:

1. members of the U.S. Congress, governors, state legislators, and mayors (increased political and financial support);
2. the Centers for Disease Control and Prevention, National Institutes of Health, and other federal government agencies (awareness and increased efforts);

NATIONAL COALITION TO ELIMINATE TUBERCULOSIS
1991 to Present

In 1991, in response to the resurgence of tuberculosis, the National Coalition to Eliminate Tuberculosis (NCET) was formed. Coalition members come from all segments of civil society including national, state, and local public health, medical professional, health care, and service organizations. The Washington Office of the American Lung Association and the American Thoracic Society serve as the coalition's current secretariat.

The original objectives of the National Coalition to Eliminate Tuberculosis included: ensure that health care providers, especially those who practice in communities heavily affected by tuberculosis are knowledgeable about the diagnosis, treatment and prevention of tuberculosis; increase public awareness, especially in heavily affected communities, of the magnitude of the tuberculosis problem in the United States; advocate for adequate public and private response to achieve tuberculosis elimination; and encourage nongovernmental organizations, especially those working at the grassroots level, to commit to the elimination of tuberculosis, and support their efforts in this endeavor.

In 1997 the NCET membership was surveyed to ascertain support for the coalition's mission and continuing membership interest in the coalition. The majority of the members continue to support the mission of the coalition. However, the majority also believed that the Coalition's objectives needed to change given the changing circumstances of tuberculosis control in the United States. For example, the majority of members ranked the first objective low, citing the fact that the Model Centers for Tuberculosis Control that had been formed would provide education and training opportunities. Members ranked advocacy and coalition building as the highest activity for the coalition, especially at the state level. Members point to the need for information with consistent messages to explain tuberculosis as a "hometown" issue to community leaders and policy makers. This can also build upon successes in states and localities in supporting tuberculosis program activities in South Carolina, California, and Washington State. The NCET is developing training and advocacy guides for use by the local members at the statehouse level. These guides are scheduled for release at the American Lung Association/American Thoracic Society International Conference in May, 2000.

3. state and local health departments (awareness and increased efforts);

4. professional societies (awareness and political support);

5. nongovernmental organizations (awareness and political support);

6. schools of medicine and schools of public health (awareness and increased efforts);

7. members of the media (awareness and political support);

8. members of high-risk populations (awareness); and

9. the general public (awareness and political support).

Key messages from this report are that even though tuberculosis is in decline, pressure to eliminate the disease needs to be increased or there will be a resurgence as there has been in the past. Issues to be addressed by the policy makers, as abstracted from the recommendations include:

• Adequate funding needs to be maintained (categorical at the federal level) and adjusted for inflation.
• State regulations mandating the completion of treatment need to be kept current.
• Regionalizing activities and using contracts with the private sector where this will enhance delivery of services.
• Providing educational resources to maintain excellence in tuberculosis services.
• Increasing resources for the prevention of tuberculosis through programs of targeted screening and treatment of latent infection, including enhanced programs focused on contacts to infectious cases, newly arriving immigrants from countries with high rates of tuberculosis, and residents of correctional facilities and other congregate settings.
• Increasing resources for research especially for the development of new diagnostic tools and treatments for latent infection and the development of a vaccine to prevent infection.
• Increasing involvement in support of global tuberculosis control through multilateral and bilateral agreements.

As has been demonstrated in the past century of control efforts, social mobilization is critical to sustaining tuberculosis control programs. Moreover, the tuberculosis control community must pay as much attention to social mobilization efforts it pays to the technical, medical, and scientific issues.

REFERENCES

Centers for Disease Control and Prevention. 1989. A strategic plan for the elimination of tuberculosis in the United States. *Morbid Mortal Weekly Rep* 38(S-3):1–25.

Centers for Disease Control and Prevention. 1999. Tuberculosis elimination revisited: Obstacles, opportunities and a renewed commitment. *Morbid Mortal Weekly Rep* 48(RR-9):1–13.

Shyrock, R.H. 1957. *National Tuberculosis Association: 1904–1954.* New York: National Tuberculosis Association.

World Health Organization Global Tuberculosis Program. 1998. Report of the ad hoc committee on the tuberculosis epidemic, 17–19 March, 1998, London.

APPENDIXES

APPENDIX
A

Statement of Task

The study will review the current state of tuberculosis mortality, morbidity, and prevention/control efforts in the United States, with special emphasis on regional and other variations; assess special challenges and solutions for the high proportion of U.S. cases of TB in foreign-born persons; and review the current state of research and development in the United States on new diagnostics and therapeutics for TB prevention, control and elimination; review the extent of multi-drug resistant tuberculosis and analyze factors that contribute to its development; and examine the role of the United States in international efforts at tuberculosis control. The committee will develop conclusions and recommendations regarding: a framework to guide a national campaign to eliminate TB in the United States; region-specific action steps required to work towards that goal; research needs and priorities for national TB elimination; information for health care providers and the public regarding the importance of vigilant and continued attention to TB control; health plan (fee-for-service and managed care) responsibilities for TB prevention and control; federal, state, and local public health policy maker's responsibilities and options regarding infrastructure needs; and strategies for U.S. contributions to worldwide TB prevention and control, leading to worldwide TB elimination.

The study will be carried out by a committee of 15 members with expertise in epidemiology, health policy, public health, clinical medicine, microbiology/basic sciences, international health, and social sciences. The slate of nominees was drawn up so that the committee would be composed, in roughly equal numbers, of nominees with extensive experience and expertise in tuberculosis issues, those with limited tuberculosis experience, and those with no significant tuberculosis experience. The completed report will be delivered to the sponsor, the Centers for Disease Control and Prevention, no later than July 31, 2000.

APPENDIX
B

Public Session Agendas

Committee on the Elimination of Tuberculosis in the United States

FIRST COMMITTEE MEETING
March 8–9, 1999

March 8 (closed meeting)

6:00 p.m.
Introduction and Overview
Bias Discussion
Clyde Behney will be leading the bias discussion.

7:00 p.m.
Dinner

March 9

8:00 a.m.
Welcome and Introductions

8:15 a.m.
Tuberculosis in the United States
Sponsor's Goals
Overview of U.S. Tuberculosis Epidemiology
Organization of U.S. Tuberculosis Control
Foreign-Born Tuberculosis in the United States
Ken Castro and Ida Onorato, CDC
Ken Castro is the Director of the Division of
    Tuberculosis Elimination at the Centers for
    Disease Control and Prevention and will
    probably present the material on the Centers
    for Disease Control and Prevention goals for
    the study and on the organization of
    tuberculosis in the United States. Ida

Onorato is the Chief of the Surveillance, Epidemiology and Investigations Branch, in the Tuberculosis Division and will be presenting on the U.S. Tuberculosis epidemiology and foreign-born Tuberculosis in the United States. In previous discussions I have asked them to avoid encyclopedic "data dumps" and to try to highlight what they see as the key issues for the committee.

10:45 a.m.   Break

11:00 a.m.   TB Research
Ann Ginsberg, National Institutes of Health
Dr. Ginsberg is the program officer for Tuberculosis projects at the National Institute of Allergy and Infectious Diseases, National Institutes of Health. I have asked her to provide an overview of Tuberculosis research in general, not just what is happening in the National Institutes of Health. I also asked her to avoid an encyclopedic list but to provide a sense of the research priorities, whether work is under way in that area, and where there are research gaps.

11:30 a.m.   U.S. Role in Global Tuberculosis
Amy Bloom, U.S. Agency for International Development
Dr. Bloom is a Centers for Disease Control and Prevention assignee at the U.S. Agency for International Development providing technical support in the Health and Nutrition Division. AID has just recently allocated funds for Tuberculosis program support and has provided limited support to the World Health Organization and I asked her to outline this for the committee.

Bess Miller, Centers for Disease Control and Prevention
Dr. Miller is Assistant Director for Science in
the Tuberculosis Division at Centers for
Disease Control and Prevention. She will be
presenting briefly in this section on an effort
by the World Health Organization to develop
a global action plan for tuberculosis. Centers
for Disease Control and Prevention is
involved in and supports this effort.

12:00 p.m.   Information Needs and Sources
                        Commissioned Studies
                        Invited Expert Presentations
                        Site Visits

12:45 p.m.   Adjourn Public Session

1:00 p.m. (closed meeting)
                        Committee Planning
                        Future Meetings

3:00 p.m.   Adjourn

FIRST WORKSHOP
June 7–8, 1999

PUBLIC AGENDA

Monday, June 7

8:30 a.m.   10-Year Review of the Strategic Plan by ACET
                        *Charles Nolan, Advisory Committee for the
                        Elimination of Tuberculosis*

9:30 a.m.   Human Rights, Social and Legal Considerations
                        *Lawrence Gostin, Georgetown University Law
                        Center*

10:30 a.m.   Break

10:45 a.m.   Population Specific Issues
                           • Tuberculosis Elimination at the United
                           States-Mexico Border
                           Miguel Escobedo, Texas Department of Public
                           Health
                           • Tuberculosis Elimination in Migrant and
                           Seasonal Workers
                           Deliana Garcia, Migrant Clinicians Network
                           • Tuberculosis Elimination in the Homeless/
                           Marginally Housed
                           Andrew Moss, University of California at San
                           Francisco

12:15 p.m.   Lunch

1:00 p.m.   Case Studies
                           • Tuberculosis Elimination, the New York
                           Experience
                           Paula Fujiwara, New York City Department of
                           Health
                           • Impact of Directly Observed Therapy
                           Stephen Weis, University of North Texas Health
                           Science Center at Fort Worth
                           • Tuberculosis in the District of Columbia
                           Michael Richardson, Medical Society of DC
                           • TB Elimination in Low-Incidence Areas
                           Carol Poszik, South Carolina Department of Health
                           and Environmental Control

3:00 p.m.   Break

3:20 p.m.   Contact Investigations and Outbreaks
                           • Expanded Contact Investigations
                           Nancy Dunlap, University of Alabama at
                           Birmingham.
                           • Managing Tuberculosis Outbreaks
                           Ida Onorato, Centers for Disease Control and
                           Prevention

4:40 p.m.   Employee Health and Institutional
                           Transmission
                           • Revised OSHA Regulations
                           Amanda Edens, Occupational Safety and Health
                           Administration

　　　　　　　　　　　　　• Staff Track
　　　　　　　　　　　　　Eugene McCray, Centers for Disease Control and
　　　　　　　　　　　　　Prevention

6:00 p.m.　　　　　　　　Adjourn

Tuesday, June 8

8:00 a.m.　　　　　　　　Tuberculosis in the Foreign Born
　　　　　　　　　　　　　• Legal Issues in Immigration
　　　　　　　　　　　　　Sophia Cox, Immigration and Naturalization Service
　　　　　　　　　　　　　• Tuberculosis Screening of Immigrants
　　　　　　　　　　　　　Nancy Binkin, Centers for Disease Control and
　　　　　　　　　　　　　Prevention
　　　　　　　　　　　　　• Tuberculosis Elimination (Screening and
　　　　　　　　　　　　　Prevention) Among Immigrants in the United
　　　　　　　　　　　　　States
　　　　　　　　　　　　　Charles Nolan, Seattle-King County Department of
　　　　　　　　　　　　　Public Health

9:30 a.m.　　　　　　　　General Discussion and Questions

10:00 a.m.　　　　　　　Break

10:15 a.m.　　　　　　　Economic Issues
　　　　　　　　　　　　　• Costs of Tuberculosis
　　　　　　　　　　　　　Zachary Taylor, Centers for Disease Control and
　　　　　　　　　　　　　Prevention
　　　　　　　　　　　　　• Securing Funding for Tuberculosis
　　　　　　　　　　　　　Elimination
　　　　　　　　　　　　　Tim Westmoreland, Georgetown University Law
　　　　　　　　　　　　　Center

11:35 a.m.　　　　　　　Modeling Tuberculosis Elimination
　　　　　　　　　　　　　Sally Blower, University of California at San
　　　　　　　　　　　　　Francisco

12:00 p.m.　　　　　　　Adjourn

THIRD MEETING
August 17–19, 1999

Tuesday, August 17

U.S. Role in Global Tuberculosis Control

8:30–9:30 a.m.	Current U.S. Activities in Global Tuberculosis Control *Nancy Binkin, Division of Tuberculosis Elimination*
9:30–10:30 a.m.	A World Health Organization Perspective on the U.S. Role in Global Tuberculosis Control *Arata Kochi, World Health Organization*
10:30 a.m.	Break
10:45–11:45 a.m.	A Nongovernmental Organization Perspective *Hans Rieder, International Union Against Tuberculosis and Lung Disease*
11:45–12:30 p.m.	General Discussion
12:30–1:30 p.m.	Lunch

Training and Education Issues in Tuberculosis Control

1:30–2:15 p.m.	Strategic Plan for Training and Education in Tuberculosis *Andrea Green-Rush, Francis J. Curry National Tuberculosis Center, University of California at San Francisco*
2:15–3:00 p.m.	Centers for Disease Control and Prevention Activities in Tuberculosis Training and Education *Wanda Walton, Division of Tuberculosis Elimination*
3:00–3:15 p.m.	Break

3:15–4:00 p.m.   Innovative Programs in Health Communication
                     *Scott Ratzan, Academy for Educational
                     Development*

4:00–4:45 p.m.   Risk Communication
                     Julie Downs, Carnegie Mellon University

4:45–5:30 p.m.   General Discussion

Wednesday, August 18

8:30 a.m.–5:30 p.m.   Closed Session

Thursday, August 19

8:30 a.m.–1:00 p.m.   Closed Session

FIFTH MEETING
January 11–13, 2000

Tuesday, January 11

8:30 a.m.–12:30 p.m   Roundtable Discussion on the Practical, Legal,
                     and Ethical Issues Related to:

8:30 a.m.–8:45 a.m.   Introductions
                     T. Alexander Aleinikoff, Professor of Law,
                     Georgetown University
                     Mark Barnes, Proskauer Rose LLP
                     Angela M. Bean, Angela M. Bean and
                     Associates Lawyers
                     Kenneth Castro, Centers for Disease Control
                     and Prevention
                     Susan T. Cookson, Centers for Disease Control
                     and Prevention
                     Sophia Cox, Adjudications Officer, Immigration
                     and Naturalization Service
                     Michael Garotte, Consular Officer, Visa
                     Section, U.S. Department of State

Andrew I. Schoenholtz, Director of Law and
Policy Studies, Georgetown University
Douglas Shenson, M.D. M.P.H., Director,
Human Rights Clinic, Montefiore Medical
Center, North Central Bronx Hospital

8:45 a.m.–10:15 a.m.   Can tuberculin skin testing be conducted for
immigrants to the United States in their country
of origin?

Can a B3 category be created for individuals
with a positive tuberculin skin test and people
in this category be processed much as category
B1 and B2 immigrants are processed now?

Can the health screening requirements differ on
the basis of country of origin?

Is the estimated prevalence of infection in other
countries a suitable criterion for deciding who
should be tuberculin tested prior to arrival?

Should immigrants from Mexico be tuberculin
skin tested prior to immigration, since
individuals born in Mexico account for the
greatest number of foreign-born cases, even
though the official estimates of the prevalence
of infection is not above the global median?

10:15 a.m.–10:30 a.m.   Break

10:30 a.m.–12:30 p.m.   Can the completion of tuberculosis screening
for immigrants with Class B waivers be tied to
the right to permanent residence in the United
States?

Should the completion of tuberculosis screening
for immigrants with Class B waivers be tied to
the right to permanent residence in the United
States?

Should the completion of treatment for latent
infection be legally mandated for individuals
with the highest risk for developing
tuberculosis?

Can/should individuals, other than immigrants and refugees, entering the United States for long periods of time, such as students, trainees, workers, and their families, be required to have screening for tuberculosis?

Could the completion of tuberculosis screening be made the responsibility of the sponsor of the students, trainees, workers, and their families?

12:30 p.m.	Adjourn the Public Session
12:30–1:30 p.m.	Lunch
1:30–5:30 p.m.	Executive Session (Closed to the Public)

Wednesday, January 12

8:30 a.m.–5:30 p.m.	Executive Session (Closed to the Public)
	Continue Review of Report Draft

Thursday, January 13

8:30 a.m.–3:30 p.m.	Executive Session (Closed to the Public)
	Continue Review of Report Draft
	Discuss Report Release and Dissemination Plan

APPENDIX
C

Site Visit Summaries

ATLANTA SITE VISIT
JULY 19–20, 1999

Committee members Donald Hopkins and Audrey Gotsch, accompanied by Larry Geiter and Donna Almario, visited with CDC staff in Atlanta on July 19, 1999. The focus of the visit was the activities the Field Services Branch of the Division of Tuberculosis Elimination. There were additional presentations on the Public Health Prevention Service and TB laboratory activities.

Field Services Branch

The Field Services Branch provides medical and programmatic consultation to State and local health departments in tuberculosis control activities and is a focal point linking the CDC with TB controllers. One current priority of the branch is enhancing program evaluation activities. Medical officers in the branch have been teamed with the public health advisor consultants to work with the State and local programs on evaluation activities. Evaluation indexes have been revised and new report forms (replacing the "Rainbow Reports") have been submitted to OMB for clearance. The purpose of these changes is to increase accountability in the use of cooperative agreement funds (see below). Don Hopkins commented on the evaluation indexes advising that a few of these, preferably only two or even one, if possible, should be chosen as milestones toward elimination.

The cooperative agreements are up for renewal this year and are based on level funding. This is actually an effective reduction in funding, due to inflation, and a real reduction in funding, since many of the program areas have relied on carry-over funds from previous years to maintain their level of funding. The cooperative agreement funding has been divided into funding for core activities (surveillance, laboratory, completion of therapy for active cases, and contact investigation) and funding for elimination activities (e.g., targeted tuberculin testing and treatment of latent infection). Five percent of the funding is reserved for the elimination activities and is dependent on the performance in the core activities.

The branch has 48 field staff positions assigned to State and local tuberculosis programs. Currently there are 33 public health advisors and 5 medical officers assigned and 12 vacancies. The medical officer assignments are considered a priority to provide additional public health physicians in the future with training and experience in tuberculosis. The large number of vacancies is a result of a CDC decision in 1994 to suspend hiring of new public health advisors through the STD and TB programs. The tuberculosis division has received approval to hire entry level public health advisors and plans to bring on 8–10 new hires.

Addressing elimination issues, the branch staff commented that level funding will clearly be inadequate. Regionalization of services and expertise will also be in important issue.

Public Health Prevention Service

The decision to suspend hiring in the public health advisor series was followed by the creation of a training program called the Public Health Prevention Service. This is three-year program consisting of one year of three-month rotations through different programs in Atlanta and two years of working in a State and local program with a CDC and local mentor advising them. Candidates for the program all have Master's degrees in a field related to public health, the third class of 25 has recently begun training, and the first class will graduate next year. This program will provide a program designed in consultation with the State and local programs for highly trained staff to assist with program planning, implementation, and evaluation.

Laboratory

Laboratory issues were addressed by staff from the Division of Laboratory Services in PHPPO and from the Tuberculosis and Mycobacterial Laboratory Branch in the Division of HIV/AIDS, STD and Tuberculosis Laboratories. The Division of Laboratory Services is involved in a variety of training and laboratory assessment activities. A major issue is maintaining training levels and competence as tuberculosis laboratory services are more often provided in the private sector. One challenge for working with the private laboratories has been developing reimbursement models so that rapid smear results can be provided on site before referring the specimen to a full service laboratory. The division is also providing assistance internationally through the development of training materials and providing consultation to selected national laboratories (Mexico) through WHO and PAHO. The laboratory provides reference laboratory services and a national genotyping surveillance network through seven laboratories. The surveillance project currently covers about 15% of isolates in 15 states. The laboratory also provides consultation in the evaluation of new laboratory technology for operational use.

The site visit on July 20 continued with a review of the tuberculosis program in Atlanta and the State of Georgia by Don Hopkins and the IOM staff.

Fulton County Health Department of Health and Wellness serves the largest county in the state of Georgia, covering a 535 contiguous square mile area and encompassing approximately 88 percent of the city of Atlanta. 187 cases were reported 1998. The vast majority were U.S.-born African-Americans with a smaller proportion of foreign-born cases than the average of the United States. Public services are provided through a central tuberculosis clinic staffed by clinic and outreach staff. Major challenges to the program include a reorganization of staffing and cost-recovery efforts. The county HIV/AIDS, STD, and TB programs are being merged in an attempt to reduce costs and enhance service delivery. The merger has just begun and management staff expressed optimism that outreach workers would be able to provide multiple services to the patients and families they work with. Outreach staff expressed some concern about cross training. No one is denied services due to an inability to pay but, after receiving services, everyone must complete an interview about their ability to pay and receive a bill. Third-parties are billed when there is insurance. Outreach and clinic staff expressed concern that, even though patients will not be required to pay, charging for services and the eligibility interview will serve as a barrier for the patients.

Grady Hospital

Grady Hospital is a large public hospital located across the street from the health department. The tuberculosis services are provided by staff from Emory University. During our meeting it was pointed out that about 25% of all cases in the State are first encountered and treated at Grady Hospital. While Grady Hospital receives about $350,000 annually in combined state and federal funding for tuberculosis activities, staff expressed concern that the public hospital, locally and nationally, is rarely considered part of the tuberculosis program or considered for tuberculosis funding. Nosocomial transmission was identified as a major problem at Grady Hospital in the past and a state-of-the-art isolation facility was constructed on one floor. One of the advantages of having the single isolation unit was that staff were better able to keep patients in their rooms and daily sputum collection could be more easily managed.

Georgia State Program

Georgia has the second highest rate among states in the southeast and 631 cases were reported in 1998, a decline from a peak of 909 cases in 1991. Two special issues discussed were management of contact and outbreak investigations and obtaining Medicaid reimbursement for tuberculosis. A report was recently published on an outbreak in Georgia associated with a floating card game. The cases occurred over a considerable period of time before it was recognized as a cluster since contact interviews were focused on households. It was only after a significant increase in cases in the area resulted in an outbreak investigation that the association was uncovered. The State staff are considering ways to train local staff who only occasionally deal with tuberculosis on ways to conduct more complete contact interviews and investigations.

Several attempts to obtain Medicaid reimbursement for tuberculosis have been made and the State Medicaid program has declined the request each time. The apparent reasons are a concern that once Medicaid eligibility is improved that the number of cases will suddenly increase dramatically (not totally incorrect if treatment of latent infection is included) and that the Medicaid budget will increase dramatically, a politically sensitive issue.

WASHINGTON, D.C., SITE VISIT
SEPTEMBER 29, 1999

On September 29, 1999, Philip Hopewell, Patrick Chaulk, and Fran DuMelle represented the IOM's Committee on Tuberculosis Elimination, and IOM staffer, Donna Almario, visited D.C.'s Tuberculosis Clinic located on the grounds of D.C. General Hospital. The site visit provided a closer look at the effects of the lack of political will.

D.C. had 107 tuberculosis cases in 1998, and it is projected that D.C. will have only 70-75 cases in 1999, approximately a 30% decrease. Officials were speculating if this decrease is true.

Funding

There has been some concern raised in the proportional decrease in funding as cases decrease. As cases decrease, there will be less DOT and fewer case investigations; however, the program cannot afford to lose 25% of their funding because of a decrease in cases.

The local government funds about 50% of the TB programs whereas the federal government provides the other half (covering staff, x-rays, and reagents). A majority of the federal funding comes from CDC's cooperative agreement, and other support comes from Public Health Block Grants. Federal funds are limited, though, in that they do not cover funds for building maintenance or medications.

The Effects of an Organization in Disarray

Several problems plague the D.C.'s TB control program: program disorganization, dilapidated facilities, outdated computer programs, and an insufficient number of staff. Most of these problems reflect the disarray and the lack of political will in the D.C. government, including frequent turnover of top officials, political officials unfamiliar with tuberculosis, restructuring within the Department of Health, and budget difficulties.

In light of these problems, steps have been taken to reorganize the tuberculosis program. Margaret Tipple, a CDC advisor, joined the program six months ago and has taken the initiative to improve the program by assuming the director's role. Unlike most CDC advisors who assist local TB programs, Tipple has taken the lead role in the TB program. Although a benefit to the D.C. program on a short-term bias, her role may not be beneficial in the long term since there may be an overreliance on the local program on CDC.

Laboratory

The impact of the political structure in D.C. has contributed to an incomplete public health laboratory renovation. In 1997, the Centers for Disease Control and Prevention granted $400,000 to renovate D.C.'s public health laboratory. After 3 years the laboratory is now 90% complete, with a new incubator and refrigerator, stocked with now expired reagents, and designed as a level 3 laboratory. However, due to the lack of trained personnel, the laboratory will remain inoperable for the next few months.

Participants at the site visit commented that it would be beneficial to have a full service TB laboratory in the District, especially given that ten hospitals and several medical schools are in the area. Tuberculosis specimens were previously sent to a Virginia laboratory, but D.C. preferred to retain the specimens. Thereafter, the TB clinic arranged an informal agreement with D.C. General to test specimens, including AFB smears, cultures, and rapid testing. Drug sensitivity tests are sent to an outside laboratory.

Housing

Two apartment buildings with four units each were available for MDR-TB cases and potentially noncompliant patients. The landlord breached the contract, and the tuberculosis program does not have housing for these individuals. The program is in the process of looking for replacement housing.

Outreach Workers

There are seven outreach workers and one manager who oversee the DOT program at the TB clinic. On average, each outreach worker supervises eight patients and visits each patient three times a week. In addition to administering DOT, each outreach worker conducts case investigations, screening, educational activities, TB skin testing, contact investigations, and brings positive skin tester in for X-rays. The staff is overworked and had problems reaching these patients until six months ago when the program acquired a car. Since many of these cases deal with multi socioeconomic issues, including being in and out of correctional facilities, comorbidity of STDs and HIV, using drugs, and/or being homeless, having a social worker on staff would be beneficial to caring for the patients.

Foreign Born

In 1998, there were 107 reported active cases of tuberculosis. Of these cases, 33% were in the foreign born. Country of origin for these cases include the Philippines, Mexico, Haiti, India, and Vietnam. The length of stay in the U.S. was the following: 24% were here 1 to 9 years, 6% were here less than one year, and for 67% of them, the length of stay was unknown. In addition, 12% were homeless and 27% were HIV-positive. Given the increase in the foreign born, it has been difficult treating them given the cultural and language barriers. There is no interpreter on staff to assist providers in caring for these individuals.

Registry

The registry for tuberculosis cases has several problems: no computer specialist, shortness of staff, numerous vacancies, and dated operating systems and hardware programs. To date, the programs were not Y2K compliant.

Partnership with TB Task Force

In response to a 1994 CDC review, the D.C. Medical Society, along with the D.C. American Lung Association established the TB Task Force to oversee the D.C. tuberculosis program. The task force meets yearly to discuss accomplishments and goals and have taken issues, such as the laboratory, under their responsibility. However, even with this organization, it has been difficult to build political will. For example, a half-day conference was recently organized to discuss goals for D.C.'s TB control program. Goals created during the meeting were produced only in an internal document and were not disseminated outside the Task Force.

Michael Richardson, head of the TB Task Force, started to establish a good control program; there should be ongoing communication between the CDC and local officials to ensure the longevity of such a program. D.C. needs continuity of leadership to promote the message about TB.

Conclusions

D.C. has problems typical of many urban centers. But because of the political disorganization of the city government, this has augmented the quality of care to tuberculosis patients in the city. These is seen in the examples cited above: the lack of staff, an incomplete public health laboratory, lack of housing for highly infectious individuals, and difficulties in communicating to a growing TB population in the foreign-born.

MASSACHUSETTS SITE VISIT
AUGUST 16, 1999

On August 16, 1999, Ronald Bayer, Sue Etkind, and Morton Swartz from the IOM Committee, along with Lawrence Geiter and Donna Almario, IOM staff, visited Boston, Massachusetts to learn from the TB control programs on both the city and state level.

Boston Tuberculosis Control Program

John Bernardo, Denise O'Connor, and Claire Murphy presented an overview of Boston's Tuberculosis Control Program. The program is located at the Boston Medical Center and is the largest tuberculosis clinic in the state with more than 10,000 visits per year. It provides resources for diagnosis and management of tuberculosis and offers free services including free medication.

In 1998 there were 89 tuberculosis cases in the Boston area. Seventy-two percent of these cases were in the foreign born, representing 52 countries. In terms of preventive therapy, language and cultural issues are seen as a barrier to administering therapy. Because of these and other issues, all tuberculosis cases in Boston are cared for under a nursing case management system.

Nursing Case Management System

In this case management model, public health nurses are utilized to assist in managing patients with various cultural and ethnic backgrounds. These issues can been seen as barriers, but the nurses work with the patients to coordinate administration of TB therapy. The main mission of the management is to promote the coordination of necessary medical, nursing, outreach, and social services to assure that all suspected and confirmed cases of tuberculosis are appropriately and effectively treated. The model attempts to maintain trust between the patient and the provider, acknowledges patients' rights in their own treatment, and assure treatment completion.

The public health nurses have the following responsibilities as case manager:

- *Clinician*. The public health nurse collaborates with the primary physician, follows patients from diagnosis to discharge, continually assesses the clinical response and treatment adherence, conducts contact investigation, and medical evaluation of contacts.
- *Coordinator of Care*. Develops and adjusts individualized management plan, Facilitates necessary collaborations to implement treatment, coordinates discharge planning from *inpatient facilities, and enforces involuntary hospitalization (last resort)*.
- *Educator*. Assesses education needs, designs education plan sensitive to health beliefs, provides TB information to families, colleagues, and community.
- *Patient Advocate*. Recognizes societal factors that impact on treatment completion, becomes a liaison between patient and social services, develops responses to address non-clinical issues, and helps patient accommodate TB treatment as a personal priority.

From 1993 to 1997, there were 469 tuberculosis cases in Boston who were alive at diagnosis and whose data were complete. A total of 401 completed therapy. The other 67 had either moved, were lost, refused/

other, or died. About 266 (67%) had self-administered therapy, 120 (25%) had total DOT, and 83 (18%) had either self-administered or DOT.

In addition the TB clinic coordinates with other satellite specialty clinics including East Boston's Neighborhood Health Center, St. Elizabeth's Hospital in Brighton, Suffolk County House of Correction, Pine Street Inn (homeless shelter), and Boston Methadone Treatment Clinics. The committee and staff visited Pine Street Inn. In 1996, there was an outbreak of tuberculosis in the homeless shelter. Since then, skin tests have been done biannually, there is a cough log, and HEPA filters have been installed. Transmission since than has decreased.

Community Based Approach Towards Prevention

Along with the case management model, the tuberculosis program utilizes a community-based approach toward TB prevention. This includes collaboration with neighborhood health centers and education of providers at neighborhood health centers. Unlike community based organizations which are federally funded, neighborhood health centers are non-profit and privately funded, with some funding from the federal government. Numbers show completion rates for preventive therapy differ between Boston Medical Center's TB Clinic and neighborhood health clinics. Neighborhood clinics had a completion rate of 80% for preventive therapy where Boston Medical Center had a completion rate of 30%.

Massachusetts Department of Health, Division of TB Control

State and local resource allocations to the cities and towns in Massachusetts vary depending on the tuberculosis morbidity rates. Instead of a county health department, each of the 351 cities and towns has their own autonomous health department. The state TB Division and the locality share responsibility for tuberculosis control. Smaller towns or areas may have variable resources to control tuberculosis. For example, Cambridge has several public health nurses, whereas in nearby Somerville, there is only one part-time public health nurse. A county health department system would help equalize resource distribution.

The Commonwealth of Massachusetts and the Centers for Disease Control and Prevention (through the Cooperative Agreement) provide a similar proportion of funds for tuberculosis control. Funds from the Cooperative Agreement cover many employees, such as central office staff, a regional nurse and outreach capacity. State funds cover the balance of the staffing, the provision of free TB medications, as well as data collection and education and training. In addition, the state provides funding for TB diagnostic and therapeutic services at no charge to all Massachusetts residents through 26 clinics statewide. Participants in the site visit commented that the future of TB service delivery may entail integrating part or all of these services with managed care organizations.

The State Mycobacteriology Laboratory conducts drug susceptibility testing on all submitted specimens free of charge. A computer system links the TB case managers with the TB Laboratory database, centrally and regionally, allowing immediate access to the most recent patient lab results. About 70% of all specimens are sent to the State Lab as either primary or reference cultures. The rest of the specimens are from managed care organizations who contract out to private laboratories within and outside of the state. This is a potential problem—specifically for quality control and cross-contamination issues.

Lemuel Shattuck Hospital, Tuberculosis Treatment Unit

The site visit participants also visited the Lemuel Shattuck Hospital which has a treatment unit used for both voluntary and involuntary hospitalization. The hospital is funded by the Department of Public Health and has a collaborative relationship with the TB Division.

SAN DIEGO SITE VISIT
AUGUST 2–3, 1999

Peter Small and Lester Wright, members of the committee, and Larry Geiter and Donna Almario, IOM staff, visited with staff of the San Diego County Tuberculosis Program in California on August 2–3, 1999 and also visited tuberculosis control facilities in Tijuana, Mexico on August 3. During the course of the visit the committee members and staff met with Dr. Kathleen Moser, Director of the San Diego County Tuberculosis Program, Dr. Sarah Royce, Director of the California State Tuberculosis Control Program, a public health nurse with the tuberculosis program in San Diego, a disease investigator/outreach worker, director of the San Diego County Public Health laboratory, a pediatrician at the University of California, San Diego, who also works with the county tuberculosis program, staff of the San Diego County ALA and the advisory committee on the elimination of tuberculosis, staff of the Cure TB bi-national tuberculosis program, and staff of the Central Health Center in Tijuana, Baja, Mexico.

San Diego is the second largest county in California and the city is the sixth largest metropolitan area in the United States. Although cases occur throughout this large city, the highest case rates are found in the downtown area and close to the Mexican border. Issues surrounding TB control in San Diego County include geographic distances, cultural and language barriers, and proximity to Mexico.

Program Structure

The San Diego County Tuberculosis Control Program is part of the San Diego Health and Human Services Agency. The program is categorical within the agency with funding from the county and categorical funding from the state. Services are rendered through a network of primary health care centers throughout the county. Health centers are located in six regions, and each region has public health nurses who provide field management services for patients in their region. Once an individual is identified as a TB suspect, the PHN case manager provides oversight until the individual until the person completes therapy, dies, etc. A disease investigator assists the PHN case managers with the most non-adherent patients. Together, they are very successful in assisting patients in completing their therapy. About 70% are on DOT. Each outreach worker has a caseload of about 10–22 patients.

Foreign Born

In 1999, there were 297 cases in San Diego. The majority of these cases are foreign-born (67%). Immigrants from Mexico and the Philippines comprise 81% of these cases.

Participants remarked on the difficulties in collaborating with the civil surgeons used by the Immigration and Naturalization Service for health examinations of individuals adjusting status within the United States. A recent study revealed that screening by civil surgeons varies in quality. A training program for civil surgeons was successful, but there is a great need for ongoing monitoring and education. It was suggested that there should be a national standardized training and certification process for civil surgeons regarding tuberculosis.

Housing Programs

The committee visited The Bissell House, a state funded housing sponsored by the San Diego County Tuberculosis Control Program and the American Lung Association of the San Diego and Imperial Counties. Non-adherent infectious patients are placed under legal orders to complete therapy. The Bissell House is used when stable housing is an issue for these individuals. Patients remain at The Bissell House until they are non-infectious, which averages between one to several months. The first infectious individual was admitted in April, 1996.

The Bissell House is comprised of three stand-alone cottages. It is surrounded by an eight-foot fence and a locked gate. About 150 feet from the house is a residential apartment that holds twelve units. Any potential issues were prevented through an aggressive program that educated apartment residents of the tuberculosis control efforts in The Bissell House.

Each unit has one bedroom, one bath, and is completely furnished. It has its own entrance that leads directly to the outdoors. In addition, each unit has its own separate air supply.

During their stay, patients wear monitoring devices to track their movement. Patients are allowed two guests at a time and they must be met outdoors. An on-site manager lives in an adjacent cottage and is responsible for cleaning and obtaining groceries.

The cost of the housing is seen as reasonable and cost-effective. The county leasing department covers utilities, the phone bill, cable TV, and food. In total, the three apartments cost the county $1,860 per month, compared to daily hospitalization costs between $600 to $1800.

Noninfectious patients are housed in rooms at the YMCA. Patients housed in both the apartments and at YMCA have been very successful in completing their treatment.

Medi-Cal

In 1994, California enacted legislation creating the Medi-Cal Tuberculosis (MCTB) program benefit. Persons with known or suspected tuberculosis infection or disease who do not qualify for full-scope Medi-Cal benefits may qualify as beneficiaries for the MCTB program.

The California Department of Health Services developed the MCTB program to provide a new funding source for TB programs to cover costs that would otherwise be borne by local communities. For persons who qualify for the TB benefit, the program covers outpatient TB services including directly observed therapy (DOT) and directly observed preventive therapy (DOPT) at $19.23 per encounter. A local health jurisdiction (LHJ) can also receive reimbursement for DOT/DOPT provided to full-scope beneficiaries. A crucial first step, however, is the ability of the TB program to enroll beneficiaries.

TB programs have encountered several challenges to identifying potential beneficiaries and enrolling them in TB Medi-Cal. Foreign-born clients often fear that enrollment in the program will prevent them from obtaining citizenship. Other challenges include the absence of a well-established working relationship between the TB control program and the Department of Social Services (DSS) or decentralized TB care systems with multiple clinics necessitating screening and enrollment at numerous sites.

Santa Clara County (SCC), through a partnership of its TB Program and Ambulatory Care TB Clinic, has been the most successful of the 49 California TB programs that meet eligibility requirements. In 1998, SCC reported 251 cases of TB; 87.6% were foreign-born Asians. SCC evaluates approximately 400 new immigrants per year suspected of having TB overseas (B notification). About 25% of the TB clinic patients qualify for full-scope Medi-Cal benefits. An additional approximately 14% are enrolled in the MCTB program. The annual budget for the TB clinic is $1.4 million.

For FY99–2000 SCC is estimating $300,000 in revenue to the TB clinic from Medi-Cal reimbursements for outpatient TB services, including DOT/DOPT. Significant additional savings are gained through direct billing of Medi-Cal for medications and laboratory services. Approximately $100,000 additional income is projected through the Health Care Finance Administration's (HCFA) Medi-Cal Administrative Services reimbursement.

SCC's success is due to several factors: two full-time TB clinic "financial counselors," a dedicated TB clinic; good marketing skills resulting in a win–win approach benefiting both patients and clinical services; development of a strong relationship with DSS; and perseverance.

The financial counselors play a key role. At the first visit each patient is interviewed regarding his/her financial status. While some credibility is gained because they are immigrants themselves, the counselors' effectiveness results largely from their knowledgeable, culturally sensitive approach. Patients are told they may be eligible for a variety of programs that will cover the cost of their care. It is clearly explained why enrollment will not prevent the granting of citizenship, and the benefits of coverage, even for non-TB conditions, are emphasized. Patients are assisted with their applications and are told to bring any bills received while waiting for approval to the counselors. It is also emphasized that no one will be denied services based on inability to pay, whether or not they qualify for Medi-Cal. The patients appreciate the concern and assistance with their financial problems.

In the face of state and federal categorical TB funding, the MCTB program has enabled SCC to expand and improve TB services. MCTB revenues are paying for the financial counselors and have helped the TB program up-grade several positions.

Relationship with Mexico

With its close proximity to the Mexican border, the San Diego County Health Department has several programs dealing with border issues.

Cure TB

Given the constant movement of individuals between Mexico and the United States, CURE TB was developed to improve continuity care for active tuberculosis patients and contacts whose care spanned the border. The program links health providers in Mexico and the U.S; informing providers of a patient's arrival to the community and by transferring patient medical information. Operated by the San Diego County TB Control Program and funded by the State of California Department of Health Services, the Centers for Disease Control and Prevention, and private funds, CURE TB also provides assistance directly to TB patients via a toll free 1-800 number accessible from both countries. CURE TB works closely with the Mexican Ministry of Health and other U.S. TB programs. As of January 2000, tuberculosis referrals were made between 24 U.S. states and 30 Mexican states. These 24 U.S. states report 90% of all Mexican-born TB patients in the U.S.

Baja California-California Binational Tuberculosis Committee

The committee provides a forum for regional collaboration between U.S. and Mexican health departments, medical professionals, and community-based organizations. The committee meets regularly and has subcommittees addressing issues of education, epidemiology, binational referrals, and laboratories. Future emphasis will be on contact investigation and binational medical case conferences.

Ten Against Tuberculosis

This initiative has been sponsored since 1996 by the U.S. Health Resources and Services Administration. Participants include health officials and CBOs from the four U.S. states and six Mexican border states, as well as federal authorities from both countries. The goals of TATB are to raise awareness of border TB issues and to mobilize strategies and resources.

Visit to Tijuana, Mexico

At the Tijuana Centro de Salud (SSA) we visited the microscopy laboratory which had a modern 2-headed light microscope in excellent working condition (provided Nov 1998 by 10 against TB), a small but clean laboratory and staff well trained in conducting un-concentrated sputum exams. Their meticulous records showing about 20 AFB exams each day. There was no ongoing laboratory quality assurance. The center was also well equipped to perform X-rays (provided in 1995 by San Diego County) and was performing 10–15 per day. A visit with the treating physician showed ample first line antibiotics being provided by the SSA, well maintained patient records including treatment cards, and a nominal registry provided by the government. A sputum induction room had been provided by a prior study and was not currently being used as it was not felt to improve the yield of un-concentrated smears.

A visit to the General Hospital (SSA) demonstrated capacity to perform concentrated smears and inoculate cultures using a Jouan centrifuge and Class II biosafety cabinet (provided by INDRE), and both a regular and fluorescent microscope (provided by "Ten Against TB"). These studies are performed on every hospitalized patient (about 15/day) and when requested by SSA clinics (5/day). Identification and susceptibility were sent to INDRE in Mexico City, but the staff shared data supporting their contention that the turnaround time was commonly too long for appropriate patient care. There was no ongoing laboratory quality assurance.

WASHINGTON STATE SITE VISIT
AUGUST 5–6, 1999

On August 5–6, the Committee on Tuberculosis Elimination visited Seattle-King County and Tacoma-Pierce County Health Departments to review the successes and concerns in controlling tuberculosis in Washington State. Patrick Chaulk, David Fleming, and John Sbarbaro represented the committee; staffers Lawrence Geiter and Donna Almario also attended. The site visit included an overview of the care provided for tuberculosis cases in Seattle-King County's TB program at Harborview Medical Center, including the DOT program, contact program, and programs targeted towards the foreign born. The committee members also visited Tacoma-Pierce County Health Department, where the public health department has been restructured to now contract TB services to a private practice, Infections Limited. In addition, the site visit group met with State Health Department TB program officers to gain an understanding of the various issues of TB control in Washington State.

In the State of Washington, the case rate is 4.7/100,000 while the case rate in Seattle is 7.0/100,000. The majority of tuberculosis cases are foreign born (67%) with most of the patients originating from Asia and Africa.

Washington State

Funding

The state motor vehicle tax may decrease in Washington State. About

$27 million from this tax went towards public health funding, $17 million of which goes to King County. During 1999 and in Seattle, the total budget of the TB program was $1.55 million: 46% was from public (via taxes), 31% was from CDC, and 23% was patient generated. Since 1993, funding from CDC has been level, and funds from taxes have decreased by about 2–3% each year (not taking into account inflation).

Seattle-King County

Overview

In 1998, 116 tuberculosis cases were reported in Seattle-King County. About 58% of the total tuberculosis cases are managed by the Tuberculosis Clinic in Harborview Medical Center. This nurse-oriented clinic has 30 people on staff.

Programs

DOT Program

In Harborview, 80% of the patients are on directly observed therapy (DOT). Each patient receives information on DOT, and Harborview Medical Center provides about half of the medication for those treated in the private sector.

Patient No. 1 A homeless patient and outreach worker provided insight into the DOT program managed by Harborview Medical Center. The patient, who is a heroin addict, was first tuberculin skin tested while in jail in 1997. His test was positive, and the jail provided him with one week of INH medication. However upon release, he was not given information on how to obtain additional INH to complete his therapy. He, therefore, discontinued therapy. In 1999, he was coughing up blood, and after a work-up, found to have a positive smear. Given that he was both infectious and homeless, he is being provided housing until he becomes smear and culture negative.

Because of the patient's drug addiction, the outreach worker provides medication daily which ensures adherence to therapy. Housing also facilitates dispensing of medication.

The patient's outreach worker commented that in terms of ensuring therapy completion and adherence there needs to be more incentives, more case management, more referrals to social services, obtaining results sooner, decreasing the size of pills, and better culture-appropriate educational material for both the patient and outreach worker.

Contact Program

Increase in funding for contact programs and cuts in prevention programs reflect that the TB population has changed from that of middle-aged homeless men, to a disease that now affects the foreign born. In Seattle-King County, one public health nurse oversees contact investigation. Thousands of contacts are reviewed, and hours devoted to contact investigation have been increased from 16 hours to 40 hours. In the recent cooperative agreement, an additional outreach worker to assist in contact investigation has been requested.

Homeless Program

One of 24 sites in the country, Healthcare for the Homeless Network is a shelter-based nursing program that refers individuals to clinical services. More than 50% are families. An outreach worker who works with the homeless individuals with tuberculosis said that trust and confidence encourage therapy completion. He notifies others in the homeless community if he is searching for someone. There is, though, a need for more outreach workers and testing of targeted populations, including injection drug-users.

Diverse Populations

Since 67% of the tuberculosis cases are foreign born, many of the TB prevention programs in Seattle-King County have focused on the immigrant and refugee population. This programming includes a partnership with community health clinics and initiating programs targeted to diverse populations. For example, Harborview Medical Center works with the International Medical Clinic, a community health clinic that offers a range of services including obstetrics, psychiatric, and acupuncture. Most of the patients are either East African or Asian. The staff is bicultural and bilingual, and physicians are trained in anthropology and public health. Suspect TB individuals are then referred to Harborview Medical Center. In addition, one outreach initiative that is designed to encourage compliance to prophylaxis treatment, specifically targets four of the largest refugee groups expected to enter the region: Bosnians, Russians, Ukranians, and Somalians. Another program, Community House Calls, targets Cambodians, Lao, Latino, Mien, Vietnamese, and Ethiopians. They serve as a mediation between Western medicine and cultural beliefs to assist adherence to therapy. For example, in the Somalian culture, sharing plates and cups during dinner symbolizes the unity of the family and community. TB-infected individuals are unable to dine in this way, and it contributes to the stigma and the ostracization of the individual from the community. Having tuberculosis is worse than having HIV.

However, there have been cutbacks in the refugee screening program. Cuts have been moved towards contact investigation.

Other Successes

Other successes in Seattle-King County include the following: no report of MDR cases in 1998, higher DOT and completion rates, and finally, number of suspect cases has increased which is being attributed to an increase in provider education.

Tacoma-Pierce County Health Department

Committee and staff members met with providers and administrators from both the Tacoma-Pierce County Health Department, the County Medical Board, and Infections Ltd., to understand the restructuring of the health department and its effect on tuberculosis services. In 1996, Tacoma-Pierce County Health Department reorganized their health department. This restructuring included privatizing the tuberculosis control program through a contract with an infectious disease specialty group called Infections Limited. Tuberculosis services, then, became part of a clinic network system instead of a categorical system.

Under the categorical system, the following were steps in caring for suspect or active tuberculosis cases (Sharma et al., draft): 1) Suspect or active tuberculosis cases are referred to the Health Department TB clinic by community providers. 2) A registered nurse would then examine the patient and a case management plan would be developed. 3) The county tuberculosis control officer, also a pulmonologist, would review all charts, order tests, examine chest radiographs, and prescribe medical treatment. 4) Public health workers would administer DOT. 5) Health department staff would report cases to the state TB control program.

With services contracted out the Infections Limited, the steps in taking care of suspect or active tuberculosis cases have been streamlined.

1. Primary care contractors notify the Health Department of tuberculosis cases.

2. The Health Department nurse epidemiologist refers suspect or active cases to Infections Limited.

3. At Infections Limited, specialty doctors would evaluate the case at the initial appointment. The health department pays a capitated rate for the care of each patient with active tuberculosis. Rates include physician and clinic visits, medications, and diagnostic tests.

TABLE C-1 Cost and Personnel Savings by Contracting TB Clinic Services

Description	Expended Amount 1996	Expended Amount 1997	Percent Change
Personnel including fringe	$384,500	232,900	39.4
General and medical supplies	$32,600	$3435	89.5
Contractual services	$60,000	$124,059	106.8
Other direct program costs	$59,300	$18,817	68.3
TOTAL DIRECT COST	$536,400	$379,211	29.3
Staffing Levels	1996 FTEs	1997 FTEs	Percent Change
Nurse	4.3	2.0	
DOT/outreach	3.2	1.8	
Clerical	1.5	0.95	
Medical office assistant	0.4	0.0	
TOTAL FTEs	9.4	4.75	49.5

SOURCE: Table provided from document prepared by Tacoma-Pierce County Health Department handout for site visit participants.

4. The nurse case manager would provide services to patients through home visits.

5. The public health outreach staff would still provide DOT.

Under the categorical system. the health department had four providers, only one site, and opened only on certain hours. Conversely, the present clinic network system now has 31 providers, 11 sites, and offers a full scope of services, 24 hours/day. Savings under the present clinic network system are in Table C-1.

In 1998, Tacoma-Pierce County Health Department reported 36 tuberculosis cases. A majority of these cases were born in the U.S. and white. Funding for Tacoma-Pierce County Health Department Tuberculosis program is $821,480 with 12% from state funds and 88% from Pierce County Special. Spending of this is as follows: 40% for TB control, 26% for TB surveillance, 7% for TB assessment, 12% for TB network, and 15% for Infections Limited.

Summary

The site visit to Washington State provided essential information to the committee. The visit highlighted the importance of culture-sensitive programs in dealing with an increasing number of tuberculosis cases in the foreign-born population, concern of maintaining funding for tuberculosis programs with potential cuts on state funding, and a new approach in dealing with tuberculosis care in low-incidence areas.

STATE OF MAINE SITE VISIT
DECEMBER 14, 1999

On December 14, 1999 Sue Etkind represented the IOM's Committee on Tuberculosis Elimination and visited tuberculosis program staff in the State of Maine, accompanied by IOM staff Lawrence Geiter and Elizabeth Epstein. The visit provided an opportunity to discuss tuberculosis services in a rural, low-incidence state. Maine has a low and steadily declining incidence of tuberculosis, but experienced an outbreak of tuberculosis at a local shipyard that involved 21 cases diagnosed between 1989 and 1992 and traced back to a single source case who went untreated for at least eight months. This outbreak generated media attention given that it occurred at a time of a national resurgence of tuberculosis. Over the last five years tuberculosis has declined from 35 cases and a case-rate of 2.8/100,000 population in 1994 to 13 cases and a rate of 1/100,000 in 1998 and then back up to 29 cases in 1999. These case-rates are well below the year 2000 interim targets for tuberculosis elimination in the United States and places Maine within striking distance of the goal of elimination, defined as less than one case per million, by the year 2010.

Organization of the Visit

The visit began with a meeting at the Maine Bureau of Health, where the site visit team received an overview of the Maine public health program and the tuberculosis program from: Joan Blossom, R.N. BSN, Director, Tuberculosis Control Program; Ellen Bridge, Consultant, Public Health Nursing; Kathleen Gensheimer, M.D., M.P.H., TB Program Medical Director; Paul Kuehnert, M.S., R.N., Director Division of Disease Control; Beth Patterson, Consultant, Public Health Nursing; Valerie Ricker, R.N., Community and Family Health; Steve Shapiro, Tuberculosis Control Program; Kim Ware, R.N., BSN, Public Health Nursing, Augusta. The primary objective of this meeting was to get an overview of tuberculosis services in the State of Maine. Tuberculosis services are provided through the Bureau of Health, Division of Disease Control. Clinical services are provided at six clinics throughout the state and staffed by TB consultants contracted by the State (there are no county health departments). One of the clinics has a sufficient caseload to operate weekly, the others are run as needed, but no more than once a month. Support for field services and patient management comes from Public Health Nursing and one-eighth of the Public Health Nursing budget is spent on tuberculosis even though only about 1% of their client population has tuberculosis. Maine provides for tuberculosis services with a combination of federal and state funds but there is a constant struggle to maintain funding. An example given by the staff of a deficiency in funding is that despite the size of the state, public health nurses are not reimbursed for costs associated with visiting patients. This is a special problem when trying to manage homeless patients, who do not congregate in one area but who are spread throughout the state and can be very mobile. There has been a particular effort to provide training for tuberculin skin testing so that case contacts, foreign-born individuals, seasonal farm workers, and others at risk for infection can be properly tested. This training is also provided by public health nursing staff. This type of training will be vital to support an expanded program of targeted testing and treatment of latent infection.

The second meeting was at the Health and Environmental Testing Laboratory, with the following in attendance: Osborne Coates, M.D., Chair Tuberculosis Program Consultants; Steve Shapiro, Tuberculosis Control Program; Julie Crosby, Health and Environmental Testing Laboratory; Joan Blossom, R.N., B.S.N., Director, Tuberculosis Control Program; Kathleen Gensheimer, M.D., M.P.H. Despite the low case-rates and the relatively small caseload, Maine retains an independent mycobacteriology laboratory. There are four full-time staff in the TB lab and in 1999 2500 specimens were processed for tuberculosis and 34 were positive. The laboratory uses genetic probes to identify TB. Federal funding supports one microbiologist and some laboratory supplies but the state laboratory budget pays for the remainder of expenses, with a charge back to the TB clinical program for TB tests. The laboratory has the objective to meet all CDC criteria for rapid turn around on microscopy, culture, and sensitivity tests. The vast majority of AFB microscopy test results are reported within 24 to 48 hours but the laboratory is not open weekends. A continuing problem is that many hospitals use out of state labs, probably due to contracts, and this delays reporting of the results to the clinicians and to the TB program. One way to improve turn-around time for samples processed within the state would be for funding to be made available for a courier service to transport specimens within the state.

While travelling to the next meeting, the IOM staff had the opportunity to talk with Steve Shapiro, a Public Health Advisor assigned to the State of Maine by the CDC. Steve works across programs, covering HIV, STDs, and TB. His background has been in STDs and his primary supervision comes from that program. His position, working across programs, is new and presents challenges in training. His focus has been on consultation in program evaluation, using CDC models. He feels that he has been able to contribute to all of the programs, that there are definitely similarities that run across all of the programs and that his ability to contribute will increase over time.

The final meeting was held back at the Bureau of Health with Kim Ware, Public Health Nursing, Augusta; Kathleen Gensheimer, M.D., M.P.H.; Osborne Coates, M.D., Chair, Tuberculosis Consultants; and Steven Sears, M.D., Vice President Medical Affairs, Maine General Medical Center. The focus of this discussion was on the role of the TB consultants. There are nine TB consultants retained by the state and paid $225 per month, plus an extra fee for each clinic session. The consultants meet four times per year and this usually provides adequate time to review all cases under care at that time. The consultants are a mixture of infectious disease and pulmonary specialists and in general feel that they have few problems managing the treatment of cases. The greatest problem was in maintaining adherence with preventive therapy. The largest group on preventive therapy are Bosnian refugees and adherence dropped as soon as they obtained jobs. DOPT has been tried in selective cases but proved not to be cost effective for their program since the number of patients in any single language/ethnic group was so small. Another difficult group to maintain adherence is seasonal agricultural workers. In general, the greatest need seemed to be to identify new strategies to deal with preventive therapy.

Before leaving Augusta, the site visit team had the opportunity to attend a portion of a meeting with the state society of the Association of Practitioners of Infection Control (APIC). There was a presentation of a complicated case that highlighted issues about skin testing, timing of discharge from isolation rooms, maintenance of negative pressure rooms, and other infection control issues. The discussion highlighted the problems faced in adhering to the proposed OSHA regulations for TB infection control. The outcome of an inappropriate patient discharge also highlighted the amount of resources consumed through skin testing and other follow-up when infection control guidelines are not followed.

The site visit team then went to Portland and met first with management of a local food processing plant and Kathleen Gensheimer, M.D., M.P.H. Two patients with active tuberculosis were identified among the workforce at this company located in Portland. The company management was very cooperative with public health in conducting screening, and later in offering work-site preventive therapy. However, company managers still felt they lacked a great deal of knowledge about tuberculosis and needed outside help to deal with the problem. Despite company cooperation with work-site preventive therapy, completion of therapy rates were very low. The major barriers included language (the employees speak a variety of languages) and the stigma the employees perceived in association with a diagnosis of tuberculosis or tuberculosis infection.

Very few of the employees understood that individuals on preventive therapy only were not a source of infection for others and education was needed in this area to make work-site preventive therapy feasible.

The final meeting took place at the Maine Medical Center in Portland with Kathleen Gensheimer, M.D., M.P.H., William Williams, M.D.; Maryann Weston, P.H.N.; and Diane Fanning, R.N. This is the largest TB clinic in Maine and is open weekly. Besides treating active cases the TB clinic works with the international clinic to conduct TB screening for refugees. About 50% of the refugees are tuberculin skin-test positive but completion of therapy rates is difficult and public health nurses make frequent home visits. Again, the problem of maintaining adherence with treatment for latent infection was a major concern. Where the medical consultants we met with in Augusta felt that community knowledge of TB was very low, Dr. Williams felt that it was very high in Portland and that he encountered few problems with poor diagnosis, treatment, or referral in Portland. This may be a residual effect of the outbreak at the ironworks and all of the attention it brought.

Summary and Conclusions

In general, the tuberculosis program seemed to be functioning extremely well and the system of contract consultants seemed well designed to provide quality care for a widely dispersed population. With the treatment of cases progressing well, there have been a number of efforts to focus on tuberculin testing and treatment of latent infection but adherence and completion of therapy are major problems. The problems the program faces are not medical but rather deal with resources. A large portion of the public health budget is going to tuberculosis and the support for this spending probably is a legacy of the outbreak at the iron works. As the memory of that outbreak recedes, the funding for the program may begin to suffer. Also, resources to expand the program from treatment to prevention of the disease are not available now and will likely be very difficult to come by.

Role of Public Health Laboratories in the Control of Tuberculosis

Robert C. Good, Ph.D.

INTRODUCTION

Awareness of what will happen if tuberculosis program efforts are not sustained, both in this country and in the world as a whole, is necessary to maintain control of the disease. Experiences from the last few years are sufficient to warn of the need to be prepared for a resurgence of tuberculosis.

There are 800 to 900 laboratories in the United States that can be classed as public health laboratories supported by government (federal, state, or local) funding (Becker, 1999). These laboratories are part of health programs that are concerned with the control of diseases, especially contagious diseases. Tuberculosis is a contagious disease that has been targeted for elimination, defined as a case rate of less than 1/1,000,000 population by 2010, with an interim target of 3.5/100,000 population by the year 2000 (Centers for Disease Control, 1989). The case rate in 1998 was 6.5 per 100,000, down 35% from the rate in 1992 (Centers for Disease Control, 1999). The data indicate that the program for the elimination of tuberculosis is being successful, and a part of the success is associated with advances made in applied diagnostics, "including new methods that reduce the time needed to detect growth of *Mycobacterium tuberculosis* in diagnostic specimens" (Advisory Council for the Elimination of Tuberculosis, 1999). The ACET has also renewed the call for the development of a new vaccine against tuberculosis. In carrying out this developmental program, the TB/Mycobacteriology Branch at the Centers of Disease Control

(CDC) should be key, establishing and using animal models to test effectiveness and safety of potential vaccines.

PERSPECTIVE

To confirm the diagnosis of tuberculosis, the laboratory must isolate *Mycobacterium tuberculosis* from the patient's specimen. This has been true since the laboratory was first able to isolate tubercle bacilli, even if guinea pig inoculation were needed to improve the chances of isolation by passage in a highly susceptible host. When specific therapeutic regimens for the treatment of tuberculosis became available in the 1950s, the incidence of the disease began to decline to such an extent that 40 years later we were able to anticipate its eradication in the United States. As quickly as the number of cases declined, tuberculosis laboratory services in diagnostic mycobacteriology became less important in the overall activities of public health and clinical laboratories. Laboratories at that time were limited to the use of the slow, but reliable, methods that had been developed over decades. Therefore, detection of acid-fast bacilli by a specific stain could be accomplished in a local laboratory or on the ward of a hospital within hours of specimen collection, but isolation of tubercle bacilli and identification based on unique characteristics required inoculation of many tubes of solid media and subcultures to measure biochemical reactions. Drug susceptibility tests also required the inoculation of a solid medium prepared with assay levels of the drugs. Results of these tests could take from 6 weeks to 6 months to complete, and during this time patients with tuberculosis were continuing to be in contact with community members, continuing to infect others by exposing them to aerosols produced by coughing and sneezing.

The laboratories responsible for tuberculosis diagnosis were not ready for the expanded workload that resulted from the increased number of cases that began to occur in 1986, when, without precedent in this century, the tuberculosis case rate reversed a downward trend and began to increase. Nor were they prepared for testing the strains resistant to multiple drugs that were isolated from nosocomial outbreaks of tuberculosis in the last decade of the century.

New procedures for the isolation and identification of *M. tuberculosis* were developed, notably the radiometric BACTEC system (Roberts et al., 1983), high performance liquid chromatography (HPLC) analysis of mycolic acids for speciation (Butler et al., 1992), molecular procedures for identification (Shinnick and Jonas, 1994), and fingerprinting techniques which provide data useful in epidemiologic studies (van Embden et al., 1993). However, laboratories were slow to incorporate the new techniques for identification and drug susceptibility testing when they became available (Huebner et al., 1993, Woods and Witebsky, 1993). Since the laboratory was limited by the slow growth of the tubercle bacillus in culture, the predominant attitudes were that there was no need to rush reporting; however, with the newer techniques, reports of identification and drug susceptibility could affect patient treatment and recovery rather than being an addendum that might be of epidemiologic significance only.

THE CHALLENGE

Understanding that a radical change needed to be made if laboratory results were to contribute to the early diagnosis and treatment of patients with tuberculosis, Tenover et al. (1993) acknowledged improved technologies available at that time and recommended that tuberculosis laboratories take positive steps to improve performance, particularly in the time taken for testing and reporting results. These recommendations are still applicable as we start the year 2000, with modification only in the addition of newer probes which can be used to probe a specimen directly. The recommendations are as follows:

(i) Promote the rapid delivery of specimens to the laboratory on a daily basis, even if this requires pickup of individual specimens to guarantee arrival within 24 h.

(ii) Use a fluorescent acid-fast staining procedure and use the time saved to immediately transmit the results by telephone or facsimile device for inclusion in patients' records.

(iii) Report patients who are suspected of having tuberculosis on clinical grounds or patients with acid-fast bacilli present on smears to the local health department promptly so that appropriate public health management (including contact investigation) can be initiated.

(iv) Inoculate a liquid medium as primary culture, and include inoculation of a slant of Lowenstein-Jensen medium.

(v) Identify growth in liquid medium as acid fast and use probes, NAP, or mycolic acid patterns to identify isolates as M. tuberculosis as soon as possible. Notify the local health department of the species identification as soon as it is known.

(vi) Determine the susceptibilities of M. tuberculosis isolates to primary drugs in a BACTEC or similar system.

(vii) Report the results of drug susceptibility testing to the clinician as soon as they are available by telephone or facsimile and follow up with hard copy. If drug resistance is present, the state tuberculosis control program should be notified promptly.

(viii) Maintain up-to-date records that include the results of quality control procedures.

(ix) Review all laboratory procedures and facilities to guarantee safety for workers.

Studies carried out on the basis of these recommendations should ensure reports of acid-fast examination of specimens within 24 h of specimen collection, identification of M. tuberculosis within 10 to 14 days, and reports of drug susceptibility tests within 15 to 30 days of specimen collection." At several points in the presentation of this challenge, reporting is emphasized. Problems arise when reports are made only to a client, such as a physician, without including notification of the tuberculosis control program. Most states specify that in-state laboratories must notify the program, but out-of-state laboratories are not covered. The notification procedures are very detailed in Title 17, California Code of Regulations, Section 2505, Notification by Laboratories for in-state laboratories and out-of-state laboratories are covered. Tuberculosis controllers, public health laboratory directors, and health officers throughout the state have been made aware of this problem, but reports may not be received from the out-of-state laboratory (Royce, 1999). When these cases are not known to the tuberculosis control program, contact studies are not initiated, and additional cases can occur.

As we go into the new millennium tuberculosis laboratories are able to isolate and identify tubercle bacilli in one to 15 days, and drug susceptibility data are available 30 days after the collection of a specimen. This level of performance is not the case in all laboratories, but in those that have actively upgraded to meet the demands for the rapid reporting of results. This ability to perform depends on a commitment to respond rapidly. Such a laboratory will have well-trained personnel using state-of-the-art methodology and appropriate equipment. The laboratory will adhere to safety guidelines and develop a safe working environment. Using up to date communications equipment (computers, FAX, telephone), the laboratory will report results of tests to aid in patient care and community disease control. These are the laboratory goals that can be achieved if specimen loads are large enough to maintain efficiency and proficiency in the laboratory.

Every tuberculosis laboratory is a mycobacteriology laboratory which is responsible for the identification of any Mycobacterium species that may be associated with a pathologic condition. Therefore, methods should be selected that will distinguish any one of the more than 71 species that have been identified (Good and Shinnick, 1998). As the number of cases declines, the laboratory is faced with the necessity of identifying the etiologic agent of a condition to rule out involvement of the tubercle bacillus, the Mycobacterium species that causes a contagious disease.

CURRENT LABORATORY PROCEDURES

Safety in the Tuberculosis Laboratory

Because of the highly infective hazard, the following steps are carried out in accordance with the recommended biosafety levels (CDC/NIH, 1999), that is, "Biosafty Level 2 practices and procedures, containment equipment, and facilities are required for non-aerosol-producing manipulation of clinical specimens such as preparation of acid-fast smears," but "all aerosol-generating activities must be conducted in a Class I or II biological safety cabinet . . . Biosafety Level 3 practices, containment equipment, and facilities are required for laboratory activities in the propagation and manipulation of cultures of *M. tuberculosis* or *M. bovis*. . . ." This requirement, along with maintenance of facilities and equipment, increases the costs of constructing and operating tuberculosis laboratories; however, the safety of personnel must be ensured. Biological safety cabinets must be inspected and certified *in situ* at least annually by approved technicians, and personnel in the laboratory must be trained in their proper use, including location, control of room air flow, placement of materials and equipment within the cabinet, and understanding of the mechanics of air flow. Safety in the tuberculosis laboratory is essential in order to prevent infection of personnel and spread of tubercle bacilli through inappropriate disposal of contaminated wastes. Details of the necessary safety procedures have been published (CDC/NIH, 1999).

Detection of *M. tuberculosis*

M. tuberculosis is one of the 22 slowly growing Mycobacterium species out of the 71 recognized or proposed species in the genus (Good and Shinnick, 1998). The number of species in the genus has increased to over 80 in the past few years as new species continue to be encountered (Metchock et al., 1999).

Specimen Collection and Transport

Sputum is the typical specimen collected for detection of *M. tuberculosis* although others, such as blood, urine or tissue, may be collected depending on the site of disease. Once collected the specimen must be delivered to the laboratory as quickly as possible. It is inappropriate for clinics to hold collected specimens to send in a batch together. Commercial laboratories have regular pick-up of specimens, and the same should be true in the public health system. This is an easily controlled step, but many laboratories have continued to use the Postal Service so that specimen delivery may take as long as a week. If necessary, public health laboratories must use a courier service to get specimens to the central laboratory within 24 hours of collection. This has not been a problem for water quality laboratories, and elaborate systems for collection and delivery have been devised by these programs that can be example for the delivery of mycobacterial specimens.

In the case of sputum, a specimen is collected on at least three, but up to five, days to optimize isolation of tubercle bacilli. If the specimen is to be shipped for any distance, the primary container is placed in a water tight secondary package and an outer package certified to meet performance tests specified by carriers (CDC/NIH, 1999). An "Infectious Substance" label must be attached to the exterior package. If the specimen is to be transported for a short distance within a building, the primary container should be placed in a water tight package and transported with care.

Decontamination and Staining

Because the specimen usually contains bacteria other than mycobacteria, it must be decontaminated prior to culture on the rich media that were formulated to promote the growth of mycobacteria in general and of drug resistant tubercle bacilli in particular. The decontamination procedures are harsh, so the steps must be carried out carefully to keep from destroying mycobacteria. The usual decontamination agent is two percent sodium hydroxide in solution with the liquefying agent N-acetyl-L-cysteine (NALC) (Kent and Kubica, 1985). Equal volumes of specimen and decontamination solution are mixed, incubated for 20 minutes, diluted to 50 ml. with neutralizing buffer and concentrated by centrifugation at 3000 to 3800 $\times$ g for 15 minutes (Metchock et al., 1999). The sediment is then used to prepare smears for staining and to inoculate various liquid and solid media. The decontamination conditions may be varied if bacteria other than mycobacteria grow on primary media, or if smear positive specimens do not then yield mycobacteria on culture.

All species in the genus *Mycobacterium* are acid-fast: that is, once the bacterial cell is stained with a basic fuchsin dye, it will resist decoloration by acidified alcohol. This very basic test does not permit determination of species, yet it is the only laboratory procedure used in many developing countries to support the clinical diagnosis of tuberculosis. The sensitivity of the procedure has been increased by using a fluorochrome stain and fluorescence microscopy. The advantage of the latter procedure, which requires more expensive instrumentation, is that the slides can be read with the low power or high dry objectives on the fluorescence microscope to observe 30 fields in about 90 seconds versus observation of 300 fields on carbolfuchsin stained slides using an oil immersion lens on a standard light microscope in about 15 minutes. In either case, the appropriate number of fields must be observed before declaring a specimen negative for acid-fast bacilli (AFB). Many laboratories that do use fluorescence microscopy do a completely unnecessary and time-consuming confirmation step on AFB-positive smears, that is, restaining using the routine Ziehl-Neelsen procedure and observation with the light microscope. This is time that could be spent in better ways.

Culture and Identification

Current Procedures

Until 1993, the routine procedure in many tuberculosis laboratories was to inoculate the concentrated specimen onto one or more slants of solid medium, such as Lowenstein-Jensen medium, which is an egg-based formulation, or Middlebrook 7H10 or 7H11 medium, which are agar-based media, and then to incubate the medium for at least 21 days at 37° C in an atmosphere of 5 to 10 percent carbon dioxide in air. When growth occurred, supplemental media were inoculated for identification of the *Mycobacterium* species using biochemical tests to determine characteristics of the strain; but if growth did not occurr, the cultures were incubated for at least 6 weeks before judging them to be negative, a criterion that is still applicable. If *M. tuberculosis* was identified by the biochemical tests, the culture was tested for drug susceptibility. Completion of these tests for identification and drug susceptibility could take weeks or months because of common laboratory practices that included batching, that is, holding specimens at various points until a sufficient number was on hand to make processing efficient.

Rapid Methods

High performance liquid chromatography (HPLC) is a rapid procedure for the identification of all mycobacteria. It was developed at the CDC to identify the spectrum of mycolic acids in the bacterial cell (Butler et al., 1992). When approximately 10^6 cells are available in culture (in 7 to 10 days), the culture can be analyzed, and within four hours the *Mycobacterium* species can be identified. The reference laboratory at CDC now uses this procedure for identification of cultures submitted, and many state and other government laboratories and universities have begun identifications by this technique. Instrumentation cost is about $40,000, but the cost for chemicals, etc., in minimal. Savings in time required to report the species can be weeks or more. The HPLC Users Group has established a

Standardized Method for Identification that is available at the CDC internet address.

Development of newer techniques to overcome the drawbacks of the BACTEC system promise to continue the advantages of rapid detection and identification. These include the Mycobacteria Growth Indicator Tube (MGIT), Becton Dickinson Diagnostic Instrument Systems, Sparks, MD, which detects oxygen utilization (Hanna et al., 1999a); the MB/BacT system, Organon Teknika Corporation, Durham, NC, which detects carbon dioxide evolution (Benjamin et al., 1998); and the LCx *M. tuberculosis* Assay, Abbott Laboratories, North Chicago, IL, which uses ligase chain reaction technology to detect *M. tuberculosis* (Ausina et al., 1997). The latter method is based on direct examination of the specimen while the first two methods are based on culture, and their performance is equivalent to the BACTEC system for detection and isolation of *M. tuberculosis*. These two culture methods are automated so that once inoculated with the processed specimen, the cultures do not have to be handled again until the time of subculture. Therefore, the advantages of the systems are decreased labor input, inclusion of a computerized data management system, use of a nonradioactive substrate, and a noninvasive technique to measure enzymatic activity of mycobacteria in culture.

The BACTEC MGIT 960 system is a fully automated, noninvasive setup for the growth and detection of mycobacteria by continuously monitoring 960 7-ml culture tubes. Hanna et al. (1999a) conducted a multicenter study to compare this system with the BACTEC 460 TB system and with Lowenstein-Jensen Medium and Middlebrook 7H11 selective plates for the detection of mycobacteria. From 3,330 specimens inoculated to all culture systems, 132 were positive for *M. tuberculosis*. The number of positive specimens detected by the BACTEC 460 plus solid media was 128 (97%), by MGIT 960 plus solid medium was 121 (92%), by the BACTEC 460 alone was 119 (90%), by MGIT 960 alone was 102 (77%), and by solid medium alone was 105 (79%). The mean times to detection were 14.4 days for MGIT and 15.2 days for BACTEC 460. These data suggest that the BACTEC 460 is the better of these two systems, but increasing concerns regarding the disposal of medium containing radioactive carbon limits its use.

Specimens can be examined directly for tubercle bacilli by PCR (Kox et al., 1997; Reischl et al., 1998; Wang and Tay, 1999; Wobeser et al., 1996), ligase chain reaction (Ausina et al., 1996; Moore and Curry, 1998; Rohner et al., 1998), and strand displacement amplification (Bergmann and Woods, 1998). In each of the studies, the particular method performed at an acceptable level, and all of them performed better with smear positive specimens than with smear negative specimens.

The Gen-Probe *M. tuberculosis* Amplified Direct Test (AMTDII), which was developed for use in sputum specimens, was compared with culture and found to have a sensitivity of 93.6% and a specificity of 97.8% (Bradley et al., 1996). However, the test was more sensitive in patients with undiagnosed disease (74.7%) than in those who were receiving chemotherapy (29.2%). Also, sensitivity of the test was 95.5% in smear positive specimens and 70% in smear negative specimens. The authors concluded that AMTDII, when used in conjunction with routine smear and culture, is a useful rapid diagnostic test for suspected pulmonary tuberculosis.

Gladwin et al. (1998) concurred with that conclusion and proposed an algorithm using MTDT, acid-fast smear, and culture for the diagnosis and treatment of immunocompromised patients with suspected mycobacterial infection.

In a comparison of AMTDII, which detects rRNA, and the Abbott LCx Semiautomated Assay, based on ligase chain reaction, Piersimoni et al. (1998) found in direct tests that the sensitivity, specificity, and positive and negative predictive values for respiratory specimens were 92.8, 99.4, 98.5, and 97%, respectively, for AMTDII and 75.7, 98.8, 96.4, and 90.5%, respectively, for LCx. With extrapulmonary specimens, the values were 78.6, 99.3, 95.6 and 96.2%, respectively, for AMTDII and 55.6, 99.3, 93.7, and 92.1%, respectively, for LCx. The level of agreement between AMTDII and LCx assay results was 78.2%. The authors concluded "that although both nucleic acid amplification methods are rapid and specific for the detection of *M. tuberculosis* in clinical specimens, AMTDII is significantly more sensitive than LCx with both respiratory ($p = .005$) and extrapulmonary ($p = .048$) specimens."

After recommendations of Food and Drug Administration Panels to approve the Gen-Probe MTD and the Amplicor *M. tuberculosis* test (Roche Diagnostic Systems), the American Thoracic Society convened a workshop to examine the data and technology, to develop a consensus addressing the appropriate use of rapid diagnostic tests for tuberculosis, and to identify future research needs and directions (American Thoracic Society Workshop, 1997). The consensus agreement from the workshop was that while these tests are a major improvement over standard techniques, there is insufficient information on their clinical and public health utility. Guidelines for interpreting the tests were advanced so that when the AFB smear and the direct amplification test (DAT) are both positive, the diagnosis of tuberculosis can be considered to be established. When the AFB smear is negative and the DAT is also negative, it is unlikely that *M. tuberculosis* will be grown from the specimen. When the results of the AFB smear and DAT do not agree, additional tests are needed. Results of the DAT tests must be interpreted within the overall clinical setting in which they are used.

The nucleic acid tests detect *M. tuberculosis* Complex, that is, *M. tuber-*

culosis, M. bovis and *M. africanum;* however, *M. tuberculosis* is by far the most frequent isolate in the United States. The true species can be discerned through subsequent isolation and identification steps that will identify the species.

In addition to the identification tests based on biochemical reactions, nucleic acid probes, and mycolic acid patterns, some investigators have been developing serologic tests, but often with poor success. Zhou et al. (1996) reported a rapid membrane-based serologic assay using the 38-kDa antigen from *M. tuberculosis*. This assay had overall sensitivity, specificity, and positive and negative predictive values of 92, 92, 84, and 96%, respectively, for sputum-positive patients with tuberculosis, and 70, 92, 87, and 79% for sputum-negative patients. Only 2% of healthy control BCG-vaccinated subjects gave weak positive reactions in the assay. However, the primary problems with the serologic procedures have been cross-reactivity with sera from patients who were infected with other mycobacteria so that the reactions were not reliable for diagnosis.

A test to measure cellular immunity was developed by Lein et al. (1999) to discriminate patients infected with *Mycobacterium avium* from those infected with *M. tuberculosis.* The test is based on in vitro gamma interferon responses by peripheral blood mononuclear cells to a 6-kDa early secreted antigenic target which is found almost exclusively in *M. tuberculosis* Complex species. Significant responses were detected in 16 of 27 patients with pulmonary tuberculosis, but the antigen was not detected in specimens from any of the eight patients with *M. avium* disease or in any of the eight healthy controls. When purified protein derivative (Tuberculin PPD) was used as the antigen, the mononuclear cells from 23 of 27 patients with *M. tuberculosis* disease, two of eight patients infected with *M. avium*, and five of eight healthy controls gave significant gamma interferon responses. This reaction is one that may be developed into a sensitive test for the diagnosis of tuberculosis, but it is not sensitive enough in its present form to replace nucleic acid tests for diagnosis.

Although nucleic acid amplification techniques appear to be rapid and accurate procedures, Noordhoek et al. (1996) found that of 30 laboratories, only five correctly identified the presence or absence of mycobacterial DNA in 20 samples. Seven laboratories detected mycobacterial DNA in all positive samples, and 13 laboratories correctly reported the absence of DNA in negative samples. The authors concluded that many laboratories do not use the quality controls that are necessary to support the results of their tests. Ridderhof et al. (1998) sent 10 samples containing mycobacterial DNA to 86 participating laboratories (47 hospital, 23 health department, 13 independent, and 2 other laboratories) for detection of *M. tuberculosis* nucleic acids. Sensitivity for the detection of *M. tuberculosis* was 97.9% for all procedures used, but the rate of false positives was high in the five specimens that did not contain *M. tuberculosis* nucleic acids. The authors believe that the failure to follow NCCLS recommendations that biological safety cabinets used for culture should not be used for nucleic acid amplification studies may be responsible for the high number of false positives. These two studies serve as warnings that should be remembered as there is greater emphasis placed on developing more rapid tests for detection of *M. tuberculosis*.

New products continue to be developed for the detection and identification of *M. tuberculosis* because of the large numbers of specimens that are processed yearly to either confirm the diagnosis of tuberculosis or to rule it out as a possible diagnosis. In addition to the direct commercial advantage enjoyed by a product that is accurate and rapid, the National Institutes of Health has provided money for research to universities and other research programs to encourage studies of the fundamental nature of *M. tuberculosis*. Technology developed through these two sources keep diagnostic mycobacteriology current.

Tests for Drug Susceptibility

All isolates of *M. tuberculosis* are tested for their susceptibility to known antituberculosis drugs so that optimal therapy will be given as soon as possible. However, knowing patterns of resistance in a community is the best guide for initial therapy since results of drug susceptibility testing will take up to 30 days to obtain. When the results are available, a clinical decision must be made regarding continuation of primary treatment or adjustment based on the outcome of the tests.

Perspective

Drug resistance is a decrease in susceptibility of a strain of *M. tuberculosis* to such an extent that it is different from wild strains that have never been in contact with the drug. However, some resistant bacilli can be present in numbers too small to affect treatment. Therefore, "Resistance on the part of the microorganisms is clinically significant when at least 1% of the total bacterial population develops at the so-called critical concentrations, that is, the weakest concentrations at which susceptible bacilli are unable to grow in the presence of the drug" Canetti et al. (1963). "Critical concentration" is further defined as follows: "For each drug it is necessary to determine the lowest concentration at which the bacilli may no longer be considered susceptible, but are to be regarded as resistant ("critical" concentration). This concentration should be determined in each laboratory according to the existing experimental conditions, on a series of so-called 'wild' strains cultivated side by side with control strains.

Under the abovementioned test conditions, the 'critical' concentrations are considered to be: 0.2 mg/ml for isoniazid; 5.0 mg/ml for streptomycin; 0.5 mg/ml for PAS; 1 mg/ml for thioacetazone; 20 mg/ml for ethionamide. If at these concentrations growth is observed to the extent of more than 20 colonies (on LJ medium with an inoculum of 2 to 10×10^3), the strain is to be considered resistant."

Changes in test medium can cause the critical concentration to change as indicated in Table D-1. In addition to the critical concentrations, other concentrations are often tested so that physicians may develop a successful therapeutic regimen. Therefore, on Middlebrook 7H10 medium isoniazid is routinely tested at 0.2, 1.0 and 5.0 mg per ml, and streptomycin is tested at 2.0 and 10.0 mg per ml. The critical concentration of a drug is always included so that there is a historical basis to determine if resistance increases in specific populations over time (Good and Shinnick, 1998).

The basic test to determine resistance of *M. tuberculosis* must provide information on the total numbers of viable and resistant tubercle bacilli present in the inoculum. Therefore, dilutions are inoculated to medium without the drug and to drug-containing medium. This has been carried over in newer tests such as the BACTEC system for determining drug susceptibility to provide information on the percent of resistant bacilli in the inoculum.

David (1970) determined that tubercle bacilli spontaneously mutate to resistance to four major antituberculosis drugs. The average mutation rates to isoniazid and streptomycin resistance were 3×10^{-8}, to ethambutol 1×10^{-7}, and to rifampin 2×10^{-10}. The mutation rate for resistance to two drugs is less than 10^{-15}. Inderlied and Salfinger (1999) discuss a special population hypothesis and the action of various antituberculosis drugs acting simultaneously to both prevent drug resistance and achieve a maximum therapeutic effect.

TABLE D-1 Critical Concentrations of Drugs Used in Routine Susceptibility Tests*

Drug	BACTEC 12B	7H10	L-J
Streptomycin	2.0 µg/ml	2.0 µg/ml	4.0 µg/ml
Isoniazid	0.1 µg/ml	0.2 µg/ml	0.2 µg/ml
Rifampin	2.0 µg/ml	1.0 µg/ml	40.0 µg/ml
Ethambutol	2.5 µg/ml	5.0 µg/ml	2.0 µg/ml

*These concentrations were accepted by a consensus of laboratories using standardized techniques. One or more susceptible control strains and strains resistant to test drugs should be tested on the same batch of medium at the same time as laboratory controls.

Current Methods to Measure Susceptibility

Inderlied and Salfinger (1999) discuss the philosophy for susceptibility testing of primary isolates and provide detailed methodology for testing, particularly for the BACTEC procedure. A liquid medium is included for the primary isolation of AFB. *M. tuberculosis* strains grow more rapidly in a liquid medium, such as BACTEC, so that the bacilli can be identified in two weeks or less, and the liquid medium is ready to use as an inoculum for drug susceptibility tests in new vials of BACTEC medium. The radioactive substrate used in the BACTEC is a disadvantage, and the radioactive carbon dioxide in the vials must be read frequently. New tests have been developed that incorporate newer methodology to provide continuous monitoring for growth without the use of a radioactive substrate or individual handling of vials (Inderlied and Salfinger, 1999).

Rapid Methods

The BACTEC MGIT 960 Antimycobacterial Susceptibility Test System (MIGIT 960 AST) was developed to overcome the drawbacks of the BACTEC 460 system. The preliminary report of a limited study by Hanna et al. (1999b) indicates through a multilaboratory evaluation that it is a rapid and reproducible system. The investigators found that the results were in "high" agreement with a proportion method.

Mycobacteria Growth Indicator Tubes (MIGIT) are available and can be used without the continuous reading system. In this case, the tubes are screened by testing for fluorescence under an ultraviolet source in a darkened room without the cost of the automated reader and recorder. Rüsch-Gerdes et al. (1999) reported the results of a multicenter study evaluating this procedure and comparing the results with those obtained in the BACTEC 460 system. A total of 441 isolates were tested for susceptibility to isoniazid (INH), streptomycin (SM), rifampin (RIF), and ethambutol (EMB). Discrepant results were obtained for three isolates (0.7%) with INH (susceptible by MIGIT, resistant by BACTEC 460TB), for four isolates (0.9%) with RIF (susceptible by MGIT, resistant by BACTEC 460TB), for six isolates (1.9%) with EMB (four susceptible by MGIT, resistant by BACTEC 460TB; two resistant by MIGIT, susceptible by BACTEC 460TB), and for four isolates (0.9%) with SM (two susceptible by MIGIT, resistant by BACTEC 460TB; two resistant by MIGIT, susceptible by BACTEC 460TB). When these cultures with discordant results were tested by the conventional proportion method, the results agreed about 50% of the time with the BACTEC 460TB procedure and about 50% of the time with the MIGIT manual system. Turnaround times were 3 to 14 days (median, 8.8

days) for MIGIT and 3 to 15 days (median, 7.8 days) for BACTEC 460TB. The difference in results from the two methods was not statistically significant. In this study the data demonstrate that the MGIT tube is an accurate nonradiometric alternative to the BACTEC 460TB system for rapid susceptibility testing of *M. tuberculosis*. This system, then, is one that could be used in a developing country where money for automation is not available.

Newer methods are being developed by using genetic probes (Martin-Casabona et al., 1997, for example) or a luciferase reporter phage (Riska et al., 1999). The capabilities that are available for study of the action of drugs on *M. tuberculosis* have expanded in the last decade, and future studies based on the initial findings should result in more rapid methods for susceptibility tests.

SUBTYPING

The relatedness of strains of *M. tuberculosis* isolated from case-patients who appear to form a cluster has depended on biochemical reactions, drug susceptibility patterns, and phage typing. For different reasons, all of these procedures were either inconvenient or inaccurate. A method of DNA fingerprinting was developed by Eisenach et al. (1988) based on detection of an insertion sequence, IS6110, in the mycobacterial genome. van Embden et al. (1993) proposed standardized procedures for this restriction fragment length polymorphism (RFLP) so that data from different laboratories could be compared. Typing has been used in a number of instances to provide additional data for epidemiologic evaluations.

As pointed out by Kamerbeek et al. (1997), widespread use of RFLP to differentiate strains of *M. tuberculosis* has been hampered by the need to culture the organism and the level of sophistication needed for typing. In consequence of this observation, these investigators developed a method which allows simultaneous detection and typing in clinical specimens and reduces the time between suspicion of the disease and typing from one or several months to one or three days. The method is referred to as spacer oligotyping or "spoligotyping." In this study most of the isolates showed unique hybridization patterns, but outbreak strains shared the same spoligotype. The procedure was found also to differentiate *M. bovis* from *M. tuberculosis*.

In a study comparing molecular markers, Kremer et al. (1999) found that the RFLP typing methods were highly reproducible and concluded that, for epidemiological investigations, strain differentiation by IS6110 RFLP or mixed-linker PCR are the methods of choice. The IS6110 fingerprint patterns have high degrees of stability (Niemann et al., 1999); however, some multidrug resistant strains of *M. tuberculosis* may evolve too quickly for reliable interpretation of strain typing results over a period of a few years (Alito et al., 1999).

The diversity of IS6110 fingerprints of *M. tuberculosis* was determined by examining isolates from 1,326 patients in three geographically separate states (Yang et al., 1998). A total of 795 different IS6110 fingerprint patterns were recognized, and the pattern diversity was similar in for all three states. Ninety-six percent of the fingerprint patterns were seen in only one state, demonstrating that most patterns are confined to a single location. The authors conclude that identical fingerprints of isolates from geographically separate locations reflect interstate transmission in the past, with subsequent intrastate spread of disease.

Many studies over the past few years have indicated the value of RFLP typing in the epidemiology of tuberculosis and for indicating laboratory cross contamination as a problem. Development of similar probes will further benefit studies of tuberculosis. As collections of data are analyzed for various areas, sites may be identified as centers for the spread of particular types. Collection of these data is only an exercise if the results are not shared with the proper tuberculosis control program for follow-up.

QUALITY ASSURANCE AND CONTROL

If there are problems that affect patient care, a quality assurance (QA) plan can be developed to define the problem, to propose changes to correct the problem, and to monitor the correction process (Sewell and MacLowry, 1999). Quality improvement (QI) as defined by these authors is a management tool used to define the customer's expectations, to describe and evaluate the processes used to provide services, and to continuously improve these processes and outcomes. QI focuses on the customers needs rather than process problems, and the customer in this case may be the patient, the health care provider, the third-party payers, or others who interact with the laboratory. Quality control (QC) includes evaluating all of the steps of a test procedure to determine if the result of the procedure is accurate. Since the methods used in the tuberculosis laboratory are high complexity tests, they must be verified regularly for accuracy and precision. Methods for verification and reliability of the tests should be included in the laboratory's policy and procedures manual.

Proficiency Testing

The Clinical Laboratory Improvement Amendments (Title 42 CFR 493.825) require that all laboratories that perform any testing of mycobacteria enroll in a federally approved proficiency testing (PT) program. In

1994, there were 2862 mycobacteriology laboratories enrolled in one or more of six PT programs approved by the U.S. Department of Health and Human Services (CDC, 1995). Approved PT programs for mycobacteriology are the College of American Pathologists; the American Association of Bioanalysts; the states of New Jersey, New York, and Wisconsin; and the Commonwealth of Puerto Rico. Of the enrolled laboratories, 2,179 reported that they performed primary culture for *M. tuberculosis*. Of these, 1,166 (54%) referred AFB-positive isolates to another laboratory for identification and drug-susceptibility testing, while 699 (32%) performed primary culture with identification, and 314 (14%) performed all tests. The break in procedures indicated by this survey slows reports of results so that the entire process of detection, isolation, and drug susceptibility testing is out of phase.

The New York State Department of Health instituted a FAST Track for Tuberculosis Testing which has been highly successful (Salfinger et al., 1998). The unique FAST Track system, which is available to all physicians who provide health care in New York, includes the submission of specimens by overnight mail, 7-days-per-week service hours in the laboratory, nucleic acid amplification and susceptibility results reported by telephone, and same day reporting by FAX. The authors also list standards of laboratory practice, turnaround times, and quality assurance.

LEVELS OF SERVICE

In 1974 and again in 1983 there was concern that decentralization of tuberculosis management services might result in decreased proficiency as laboratories received fewer specimens for processing. Currently that fear is again surfacing as the number of tuberculosis cases continues to decline. Certainly, laboratory expertise will also decline if an adequate number of specimens is not processed to maintain laboratory efficiency. The laboratory that does not receive many specimens will lose financial support and will be in even greater decline.

The American Thoracic Society (1983) published Levels of Laboratory Service as a guide for referral of specimens. The original concept of having three levels of service has been debated, as well as prescribing the number of specimens that must be processed to maintain proficiency. The Level I Laboratory is to collect good specimens and ship to a higher level laboratory for culture. Level I laboratories may perform microscopic examination. If the Level I laboratory prepares and examines smears, then 10 to 15 specimens per week must be examined to maintain proficiency. The Level II Laboratory performs the same functions as Level I but also isolates organisms in culture, identifies *Mycobacterium tuberculosis*, and performs susceptibility tests. Other mycobacterial isolates are referred to Level III for identification. Level III performs all procedures of Level I, identifies all mycobacteria, and performs susceptibility tests.

The Association of State and Territorial Public Health Laboratory Directors (ASTPHLD, now known as the Association of Laboratory Directors or ALD) in their second conference on the laboratory aspects of tuberculosis in 1995 proposed that in the new age of technology only two Levels of service should be recognized (Warren and Cordts, 1996). In this classification, Level I laboratories, housed in a Biosafety Level II facility, are those that arrange for transport of specimens for arrival in their laboratory within 24 hours of collection. The Level I laboratory may prepare acid-fast smears from concentrated specimens and examine them by fluorescent microscopy so that a report can be issued within 24 hours of receipt. If the laboratory chooses to stain specimens, it shall process at least 20 smears per week to maintain proficiency, with collection and transport of specimens for arrival in the laboratory within 24 hours of collection. Level I laboratories arrange for rapid transport of specimens to Level II laboratories for processing.

Level II laboratories processing at least 25 specimens per week will perform all the following tasks and must have a facility for Biosafety level III practices. Laboratories at this level must be able to perform the following:

A. Prepare acid-fast bacilli smears from concentrated specimens and examine them by fluorescent microscopy within 24 hours of receipt.

B. Use a combination of liquid and solid media for primary isolation of mycobacteria.

C. Identify all *Mycobacterium* species using rapid methods (such as DNA probes or high-performance liquid chromatography) to ensure identification within 10–14 days.

D. Perform susceptibility testing of *M. tuberculosis* to ensure reporting results within 15–30 days of specimen collection, by either implementation of the direct susceptibility test on agar plates (especially for new patients) or implementation of an indirect test in a liquid medium.

The levels of service concept is acceptable today. The ASTPHLD levels should be considered as guidelines until a more comprehensive program is in place. The processing of specimens in two different laboratories should be discouraged because of all of the time that is lost in shipment. A Level I laboratory may serve as an information source to direct specimens to the Level II laboratory.

TRAINING

Excellence in the laboratory comes from a permanent, well-trained staff who have pride in their performance. In my view, the Mycobacteriology Laboratory should not be included in the rotation exercises found in many diagnostic laboratories because of the expertise that is demanded in test performance, interpretation of results, and the requirement for performance under the safety codes for the protection of self and others.

Clinical Laboratories Improvement Amendment of 1988

Tests for staining, isolation, identification, drug susceptibility testing, and special tests for epidemiologic studies of tuberculosis are all considered complex tests in the Clinical Laboratory Improvement Amendments (CLIA), Code of Federal Regulations, Chapter IV. Subpart M defines the qualifications of personnel for high complexity testing in paragraph 493.1489, that is, personnel should have a medical degree or "Have earned a doctoral, master's or bachelor's degree in a chemical, physical, biological or clinical laboratory science, or medical technology from an accredited institution;" or "Have earned an associate degree in a laboratory science, or medical laboratory technology from an accredited institution or" meet one or more other requirements that indicate acquisition of the individual skills required for performing specific laboratory tests, for proper instrument use, for performing preventive maintenance, and for calibration procedures." Personnel must also "have the skills required to implement quality control policies and procedures of the laboratory;" have "an awareness of the factors that influence test results;" and have "the skills required to assess and verify the validity of patient test results through the evaluation of quality control values before reporting patient test results." Qualifications of technologists as high complexity testing personnel under paragraph 1489(b)(3) are given in paragraph 493.1491. In summary, personnel performing the high complexity tests of the tuberculosis laboratory must have a level of training, preferably at least a bachelor's degree from an accredited institution, that indicates the comprehension and responsibility adequate for testing and reporting results of a critical nature.

In addition of the qualifications prescribed by CLIA, many states have criteria that personnel in the tuberculosis laboratory must meet. The local requirements mean that personnel in a commercial testing laboratory may not be able to transfer to a state laboratory even though they meet the CLIA requirements. State laboratories are obligated to work within the laws of their jurisdictions until those laws are changed.

Types of Training

Training should be available as an ongoing function of the laboratory through a collection of texts, reprints, and self-help documents, and through specific guidance by senior personnel. Outside training is available through the American Society for Microbiology (ASM), the Centers for Disease Control and Prevention (CDC), ALD, and the National Laboratory Training Network (NLTN) which is cosponsored by the ADL and CDC. The NLTN gives training courses applicable to the tuberculosis laboratory and in other clinical, environmental, and public health topics. Participation in these courses awards continuing educational credits to participants who successfully complete training.

All personnel should be encouraged to attend at least one training meeting per year, and be given as much support as possible to do so, such as compensated leave, support for travel and per diem, training fees, etc. An ongoing training program will pay dividends in maintaining an aware and capable staff. The excitement we experience in work activities is dependent on our ability to understand and interpret them.

Need for Training

CDC recently surveyed 43 state public health laboratories, 8 nonstate public health laboratories, 87 hospital laboratories, and 7 commercial laboratories to get a first line response on what is perceived to be the training programs that would best serve their needs (Bird, 1999). Although the results are in the preliminary stages of analysis, some needs stand out. Most respondents believed that additional training was needed in safety, specifically in accident response, risk assessment, and effective use of the biological safety cabinet. Many respondents also believed management training was needed for quality assurance, CLIA standards, cost effectiveness and electronic reporting. Specific laboratory problems that respondents wanted addressed were the detection and prevention of false-positive reactions for *M. tuberculosis*, training in the use and interpretation of direct identification kits for specimens that are AFB positive, and training and possible research with the advanced technologies such as PCR and RFLP. Additional training is currently being planned by the Division of Laboratory Systems, Public Health Practice Program Office, CDC, to meet these needs.

RESEARCH

Every laboratory can benefit by having a program of applied research to accompany the routine work load. Many research studies can concentrate on method development in conjunction with trials of new products, resolving cases of cross-contamination, or investigation of local clusters of disease in collaboration with epidemiologists. Studies conducted by public health laboratories may concentrate on the background and follow-up of cases of disease due to *Mycobacterium* species other than *M. tuberculosis*, particularly using the Public Health Laboratory Information System (PHLIS) that is available to them from CDC. This system allows study of all mycobacterial isolates and drug susceptibility patterns by a number of parameters. Studies of the occurrence of these acid-fast bacteria and the diseases they cause are within the scope of the tuberculosis laboratory since many of the methods will be the same and, in general, information found with one species is helpful in understanding another. Studies to discover an environmental source for these infections would be interesting. A review of data reported by state laboratories to PHLIS can be found in an electronic publication (W. R. Butler and J. T. Crawford. Nontuberculous Mycobacteria Reported to the Public Health Laboratory Information System by State Public Health Laboratories, United States, 1993–1996, which can be accessed on http://www/cdc.gov/ncidod/dastlr/mycobacteriology.htm). Additional data on the isolation of *M. tuberculosis* and results of drug susceptibility tests are not included in this report; however, each state has that information available to them, also.

Research projects should fit the interest of the investigator, but they should be of such a nature that an audience of peers will find the study informative. Development of an interest in one or more of the technologies available to the investigator may lead to discovery of a unique use that was not previously considered.

ROLE OF COMMERCIAL LABORATORIES AND THEIR RELATIONSHIP TO THE PUBLIC HEALTH LABORATORY

Public health laboratories are not in conflict with commercial laboratories; indeed, commercial laboratories do many things well that the public health laboratory needs to emulate; for example, the rapid pick-up of specimens (courier) and the rapid processing that is usually available from commercial laboratories. Many public health laboratories still depend on specimens that are held until a predetermined shipment size is reached, and are then placed in the mail for delivery by the U.S. Postal Service, resulting in a delay of several days. Public health laboratories submit reports to the client and to the tuberculosis program at stages of processing. In contrast, the commercial laboratory always sends a report to the client who submitted the specimen, but they may not always include notification to the health department (Royce, 1999).

McDade and Hughes (1998) point out that the failure of health care providers to submit representative isolates of etiologic agents to public health authorities for confirmation and subtyping will preclude the prompt identification of disease outbreaks. Public health laboratory programs are even more compromised in their attempts to discover and control infectious diseases when out-of-state laboratories fail to comply with the reporting requirements. When the tuberculosis program is not notified of laboratory results, control measures are not activated, and contact cases may be lost to early treatment.

Skeels (1999) indicates two ways that private sector clinical laboratories contribute to public health efforts: (i) by diagnosing and reporting communicable diseases and (ii) by working with public health laboratories for the referral, confirmation, and typing of microbial isolates. He also reports that many clinical microbiology directors are no longer allowed by managed care organizations (MCOs) to perform "extra" testing on patient specimens for public health purposes that go beyond the needs of individual patient care. Decisions to do such testing are now made by administrators and insurers who require "critical path management" of patients, often with the view that public health testing is an unnecessary added cost. Skeels (1999) also discusses the findings of a study by the Lewin Group, which was commissioned by the Office of the Assistant Secretary for Planning and Evaluation, U.S. Department of Health and Human Services, as part of ongoing research regarding public health infrastructure. The Group reported that managed care and other health system changes are having negative effects on public health laboratories, making it more difficult for them to fulfill their public health mission.

Costs for diagnostic services vary widely between commercial and public health laboratories in that many of the latter do not charge for specimens submitted for study. However, some public health laboratories charge more than commercial laboratories, which must realize a profit. In answer to a survey question submitted to laboratory directors in preparation for this report, only eight of 45 state public health laboratory directors, but two of three territorial laboratory directors, indicated that they charged for tuberculosis laboratory diagnosis.

Dr. Leonid Heifets at the National Jewish Hospital in Denver is the head of an active charge-for-service, tuberculosis referral laboratory. The price for an AFB smear and inoculation of four units of medium (including BACTEC) for isolation of mycobacteria is $58.00. Prices for identification vary: $150.00 for an amplification test (MTD) with a raw specimen; $49.50 for the Gen-Probe test of a grown culture (including confirmation as *M. tuberculosis* and not another member of the *M. tuberculosis* Complex) with four biochemical tests; $30.75 for a conventional identification if it is ordered along with a drug-susceptibility test. Costs for susceptibility tests are not available at this time.

Because new arrangements are needed to identify specific functions of public- and private-sector laboratories, facilitate collaboration in areas of shared responsibility, and prevent unnecessary duplication of services, McDade and Hausler (1998) proposed the formation of local public health institutes to improve the strategic planning for public health. They further assigned certain functions to public and private sectors and identified a group of functions that are shared. There are advantages that will accrue from performance under this system that should be considered, chiefly that the role of each type of laboratory is clarified in an overall planned program that can be integrated on a local or regional level.

THE POTENTIAL ROLE OF REGIONAL LABORATORIES TO AUGMENT PROCEDURES OF STATE AND LOCAL LABORATORIES

As the number of cases of tuberculosis declines, work load in the laboratory will decrease even though there are an average of 20,621 isolates of nontuberculous mycobacteria identified per year by reporting state laboratories (W. R. Butler and J. T. Crawford, Nontuberculous Mycobacteria Reported to the Public Health Laboratory Information System by State Public Health Laboratories, United States, 1993–1996, which can be accessed on http://www/cdc.gov/ncidod/ dastlr/ mycobacteriology.htm). If the trend continues, the number of isolations by some laboratories may be too rare to maintain their efficiency.

The concept of regionalized laboratories for fingerprinting isolates of *M. tuberculosis* is a potential model that can be used to increase the efficiency of public health tuberculosis laboratories. As noted above, the ATS and the ASTPHLD (ALD) endorse using laboratory activity extrapolated from the numbers of specimens processed as a guide for maintaining proficiency, over and above participation in a PT program. Use of genetic probes will not guarantee that other sophisticated procedures, such as drug susceptibility testing, are carried out for the characterization of bacilli identified as *M. tuberculosis* Complex. In areas where few specimens are processed for isolation and identification of *M. tuberculosis,* efficient use of funds and accuracy of reports mandate a regionalization of public health laboratories. Commercial laboratories have already established centralized laboratories in regions for various activities. The same approach will have to be used for public health laboratories as the number of specimens processed dwindles, because of the reduced number of cases.

Because of the sensitive nature of regionalization and the political ramifications in each locality, the problem should be considered in a special committee of the ALD. The people most involved in the problem can make the fairest appraisal of a solution.

FUNDING, GRANTS, CHARGES FOR SERVICE

State public health laboratories have received supplemental federal funding through CDC for several years to obtain equipment, to train laboratory personnel, to upgrade the level of effort needed to keep equipment and personnel current with new technology, and to develop the sophistication of the modern mycobacteriology laboratory in all of its aspects. The funding is on a five-year cycle and applications will be reviewed in 1999 for the next five-year cycle. Funding for the laboratories has been about eight million dollars per year. An additional eight hundred thousand dollars has supported the RFLP typing program.

Hospital and clinical laboratories develop relationships with commercial laboratories that may charge less for processing specimens than their state public health laboratory. Although the commercial laboratory is able to study specimens and report results in an efficient way in most instances, they should abide by the regulations of the state where specimens originate to ensure that reporting requirements for reportable diseases are all met (Skeels, 1999).

ROLE OF THE MYCOBACTERIOLOGY LABORATORY AT THE CENTERS FOR DISEASE CONTROL

The TB/Mycobacteriology Branch, Division of AIDS, STD, and TB Laboratory Research, NCID, CDC is central to the laboratory activities throughout the country. It is the ultimate reference laboratory to solve problems with difficult cultures and tests; to provide the background information through presentations, publications, and consultations on new and upcoming techniques applicable to the field; and to interact closely with the Division of Tuberculosis Elimination to support studies, give guidance regarding laboratory capabilities, and provide general back-up for their programs.

The activities of the CDC laboratory could be increased if funding were more available. Laboratory personnel need to attend meetings and conferences, many overseas. Practical research programs in the Branch need to be expanded to include studies in animals. This laboratory should be the central site to evaluate and measure the parameters of new vaccines that are being developed, but adequate animal quarters are not available for the work. The Branch should be in better contact with the state laboratories, and a good way to promote interaction would be to have the Branch, with a staff to monitor and supervise the expenditures, control funding for state laboratories.

The TB/Mycobacteriology Branch has active programs under way, and these are fully supported. The Branch has been providing training to underdeveloped countries in collaboration with other segments of CDC; however, work in these areas has been at a rather low level since the programs are in other centers and divisions. The Branch should award training scholarships to offset per diem expenses of short term trainees from this country and abroad, and support travel and per diem for distinguished scientists. If the TB/Mycobacteriology Branch is to impact studies in developing countries, direct relationships must be established, and all support activities must be through the Branch Chief with his/her assignment of the most appropriate personnel for each project.

CURRENT STATUS OF PUBLIC HEALTH TUBERCULOSIS LABORATORIES

Tenover et al. (1993) issued a challenge to tuberculosis laboratories because available technologies were not being used to speed reports of results from tuberculosis laboratories. What is the status of laboratories in 1999?

Since 1993, tuberculosis laboratories, both in hospitals (Tokars et al., 1996) and state public health facilities (Bird et al., 1996; Denniston et al., 1997; Huebner et al., 1993), have worked to upgrade their facilities and procedures. The state laboratories have been very aggressive in a program of modernization.

In preparation of this report, questionnaires were sent to laboratory directors in all of the states, the District of Columbia, and the territories. Even though the turnaround time for submitting replies was short, 46 state laboratory (SL) directors and 4 directors of territorial laboratories (TL) responded (see Table D-2). All respondents accepted specimens for the laboratory diagnosis of tuberculosis, and all processed the specimens in-house except for two TLs that sent specimens to the SLs in Hawaii and California. Replies indicated that state and territorial laboratories have updated procedures to speed identification and drug susceptibility testing. As indicated by the responses, public health laboratories are using the modern procedures available to them, and reports are being made to state tuberculosis programs in a timely manner. Since this survey did not include any of hospital or commercial laboratories, a conclusion regarding their performance cannot be made.

In the past the ASTPHLD and various Centers of the CDC have co-sponsored meetings to update the role of tuberculosis laboratories. These meetings should continue as the technology for methods of identification and drug susceptibility testing continues to develop. Tuberculosis laboratories that process initial specimens are now in a good position, but maintaining the laboratories as a first-line weapon for the elimination of tuberculosis in the United States is a major challenge that must be met.

TABLE D-2 Current Practices of Public Health Tuberculosis Laboratories

Activity	States	Territories	Total
Number surveyed	51[a]	7	58
Number responding	46 (90%)	4 (57%)	50 (86%)
Accept TB specimens	46 (100%)	4 (100%)	50 (100%)
Process in-house[b]	46[b] (100%)	2[b] (50%)	48[b] (96%)
Receive specimens within 24 hrs	23 (50%)	2 (100%)	25 (52%)
Use fluorescent AFB stain	46 (100%)	2 (100%)	48 (100%)
Report results of stain to program	45 (98%)	2 (100%)	47 (98%)
Inoculate specimen to liquid medium	45 (98%)	2 (100%)	47 (98%)
Acid-fast stain of growth in liquid medium	46 (100%)	2 (100%)	48 (100%)
Use DNA probe to identify growth	36[c] (78%)	2 (100%)	38 (79%)
Use HPLC to identify growth	6[c] (13%)	0 (0%)	6 (12%)
Notify TB program as soon as identity is known	44 (96%)	2 (100%)	46 (96%)
Determine drug susceptibility in Bactec or similar instrument	44 (96%)	2 (100%)	46 (96%)
Report results of drug tests by telephone/fax and follow up with hard copy	42 (91%)	2 (100%)	44 (92%)
Maintain current records of QC	46 (100%)	2 (100%)	48 (100%)
Review procedures/facilities for safety	45 (98%)	2 (100%)	47 (98%)

[a]Includes District of Columbia.

[b]Base number of laboratories for measuring activities that follow. Two territorial laboratories send their specimens to state laboratories for further processing.

[c]Several laboratories indicated a change from DNA probe to HPLC within the next several months.

REFERENCES

Advisory Council for the Elimination of Tuberculosis. 1999. Tuberculosis elimination revisited: obstacles, opportunities, and a renewed commitment. MMWR 48(RR09):1–13.

Alito, A., N. Morcillo, S. Scipioni, A. Dolmann, M. I. Romano, A. Cataldi, and D. van Soolingen. 1999. The IS6110 restriction fragment length polymorphism in particular multidrug-resistant *Mycobacterium tuberculosis* strains may evolve too fast for reliable use in outbreak investigation. *J. Clin. Microbiol.* 37:788–791.

American Thoracic Society. 1983. Levels of laboratory services for mycobacterial diseases: Official Statement of the American Thoracic Society. *Am. Rev. Respir. Dis.* 128:213.

American Thoracic Society Workshop. 1997. Rapid diagnostic tests for tuberculosis: what is the appropriate use? *Am. J. Respir. Crit. Care Med.* 155:1804–1814.

Ausina, V., F. Gamboa, E. Gazapo, J. M. Manterola, J. Lonca, L. Matas, J. R.Manzano, C. Rodrigo, P. J. Cardona, and E. Padilla. 1997. Evaluation of the semiautomated Abbott LCx *Mycobacterium tuberculosis* assay for direct detection of *Mycobacterium tuberculosis* in respiratory specimens. *J. Clin. Microbiol.* 35:1996–2002.

Becker, S. 1999. Personal communication.

Benjamin, Jr., W. H., K. B. Waites, A. Beverly, L. Gibbs, M. Waller, S. Nix, S. A. Moser, and M. Willert. 1998. Comparison of the MB/BacT system with a revised antibiotic supplement kit to the BACTEC 460 system for detection of mycobacteria in clinical specimens. *J. Clin. Microbiol.* 36:3234–3238.

Bergmann, J. S., and G. L. Woods. 1998. Clinical evaluation of the BD ProbeTec Strand Displacement Amplification Assay for rapid diagnosis of tuberculosis. *J. Clin. Microbiol.* 36:2766–2768.

Bird, B. R., M. M. Denniston, R. E. Huebner, and R. C. Good. 1996. Changing practices in mycobacteriology: a follow-up survey of state and territorial public health laboratories. *J. Clin. Microbiol.* 34:554–559.

Bird, B. R. 1999. Personal communication.

Bradley, S. P., S. L. Reed, and A. Catanzaro. 1996. Clinical efficacy of the amplified *Mycobacterium tuberculosis* direct test for the diagnosis of pulmonary tuberculosis. *Am. J. Respir. Crit. Care Med.* 153:1606–1610.

Butler, W. R., I. Thiebert, and J. O. Kilburn. 1992. Identification of *Mycobacterium avium* complex strains and some similar species by high-performance liquid chromatography. *J. Clin. Microbiol.* 30:2698–2704.

Canetti, G., S. Froman, J. Grosset, P. Hauduroy, M. Lagerova, H. T. Mahler, G. Meissner, D. A. Mitchison, and L. Sula. 1963. Mycobacteria: laboratory methods for testing drug sensitivity and resistance. *Bull. W. H. O.* 29:565–578.

Centers for Disease Control. 1989. A strategic plan for the elimination of tuberculosis in the United States. MMWR 38 (Suppl. No. S-3):1–25.

Centers for Disease Control. 1995. Laboratory practices for diagnosis of tuberculosis— United States, 1994. MMWR 44:587–590.

Centers for Disease Control. 1999. Progress Toward the elimination of tuberculosis—United States, 1998. MMWR 48:732–736.

Centers for Disease Control and Prevention and National Institutes of Health. 1999. *Biosafety in Microbiological and Biomedical Laboratories,* J. Y. Richmond and R. W. McKinney, eds. 4th ed. U.S. Government Printing Office, Washington, D.C., pp. 104–106, 201–202, 216–219.

David, H. L. 1970. Probability distribution of drug-resistant mutants in unselected populations of *Mycobacterium tuberculosis. Appl. Microbiol.* 20:810–814.

Denniston, M. M., B. R. Bird, and K. A. Kelley. 1997. Contrast of survey results between state and a cohort of nonstate mycobacteriology laboratories: changes in laboratory practices. *J. Clin. Microbiol.* 35:422–426.

Eisenach, K. D., J. T. Crawford, and J. H. Bates. 1988. Repetitive DNA sequences as probes for *Mycobacterium tuberculosis. J. Clin. Microbiol.* 26:2240–2245.

Gladwin, M. T., J. J. Plorde, and T. R. Martin. 1998. Clinical application of the *Mycobacterium tuberculosis* direct test: case report, literature review, and proposed clinical algorithm. *Chest* 114:317–323.

Good, R. C., and T. M. Shinnick. 1998. *Mycobacterium,* pp. 549–576. *In:* A. Balows and B. I. Duerden (eds.), *Topley & Wilson's Microbiology and Microbial Infections,* 9th ed., vol. 2, Systematic Bacteriology. Oxford University Press, Inc., New York,

Hanna, B. A., A. Ebrahimzadeh, L. B. Elliott, M. A. Morgan, S. M. Novak, S. Rüsch-Gerdes, M. Acio, D. F. Dunbar, T. M. Holmes, C. H. Rexer, C. Savthyakumar, and A. M. Vannier. 1999a. Multicenter Evaluation of the BACTEC MGIT 960 System for recovery of mycobacteria. *J. Clin. Microbiol.* 37:748–752.

Hanna, B. A., A. Ebrahimzadeh, G. E. Pfyffer, F. Palicova, C. H. Rexer, T. Sanchez, C. Sathyakumar, and L. B. Heifets. 1999b. Evaluation of the BACTEC MGIT 960 antimycobacterial susceptibility test. Abstract, paper 864, 39th ICAAC, San Francisco, Ca., Sept 26–29, 1999.

Huebner, R. E., R. C. Good, and J. I. Tokars. 1993. Current practices in mycobacteriology: results of a survey of state laboratories. *J. Clin. Microbiol.* 31:771–775.

Inderlied, C. B., and M. Salfinger. 1999. Antimycobacterial agents and susceptibility tests, pp. 1601–1623. *In:* P. R. Murray, E. J. Baron, M. A. Pfaller, F. C. Tenover, and R. H. Yolken (eds.), *Manual of Clinical Microbiology*, 7th ed. ASM Press, Washington, D.C.

Kamerbeek, J., L. Shouls, A. Kolk, M. van Agterveld, D. van Soolingen, S. Kuijper, A. Bunschoten, H. Molhuizen, R. Shaw, M. Goyal and J. van Embden. 1997. Simultaneous detection and strain differentiation of *Mycobacterium tuberculosis* for diagnosis and epidemiology. *J. Clin. Microbiol.* 35:907–914.

Kent, P.T., and G. P. Kubica. 1985. *Public Health Mycobacteriology: A Guide for the Level III Laboratory.* Centers for Disease Control, U.S. Department of Health and Human Services, Atlanta, Georgia.

Kox, L. F., H. M. Jansen, S. Kuijper, and A. H. Kolk. 1997. Multiplex PCR assay for immediate identification of the infecting species in patients with mycobacterial disease. *J. Clin. Microbiol.* 35:1492–1498.

Kremer, K., D. van Soolingen, R. Frothingham, W. H. Haas, P. W. M. Hermans, C. Martin, P. Palittapongarnpim, B. B. Plikaytis, L. W. Riley, M. A.Yakrus, J. M. Musser, and J. D. A. van Embden. 1999. Comparison of methods based on different molecular epidemiological markers for typing of *Mycobacterium tuberculosis* complex strains: interlaboratory study of discriminatory power and reproducibility. *J. Clin. Microbiol.* 37:2607–2618.

Lein, A. D., C. F. von Reyn, P. Ravn, C. R. Horsburgh, Jr., L. N. Alexander, and P. Andersen. 1999. Cellular immune responses to ESAT-6 discriminate between patients with pulmonary disease due to *Mycobacterium avium* complex and those with pulmonary disease due to *Mycobacterium tuberculosis. Clin. Diagn. Lab. Immunol.* 6:606 609.

Martin-Casabona, N., D. X. Mimó, T. González, J. Rossello, and L. Arcalis. 1997. Rapid method for testing susceptibility of *Mycobacterium tuberculosis* by using DNA probes. *J. Clin. Microbiol.* 35:2521–2525.

McDade, J. E., and W. J. Hausler, Jr. 1998. Modernization of public health laboratories in a privatization atmosphere. *J. Clin. Microbiol.* 36:609–613.

McDade, J. E., and J. M. Hughes. 1998. The U.S. needs a national laboratory system. *U.S. Medicine* 34:9.

Metchock, B. G., F. S. Nolte, and R. J. Wallace, Jr. 1999. *Mycobacterium*, pp. 399–437. *In:* P. R. Murray, E. J. Baron, M. A. Pfaller, F. C. Tenover, and R. H. Yolken (eds.), *Manual of Clinical Microbiology,* 7th ed. ASM Press, Washington, D.C.

Moore, D. F., and J. I. Curry. 1998. Detection and identification of *Mycobacterium tuberculosis* directly from sputum sediments by ligase chain reaction. *J. Clin. Microbiol.* 36:1028–1031.

Niemann, S., E. Richter, and S. Rüsch-Gerdes. 1999. Stability of *Mycobacterium tuberculosis* IS6110 fragment length polymorphism patterns and spoligotypes determined by analyzing serial isolates from patients with drug-resistant tuberculosis. *J. Clin. Microbiol.* 37:409–412.

Noordhoek, G. T., J. D. van Embden, and A. H. Kolk. 1996. Reliability of nucleic acid amplification for the detection of *Mycobacterium tuberculosis*: an international collaborative quality control study among 30 laboratories. *J. Clin. Microbiol.* 34:2522–2525.

Piersimoni, C., A. Callegaro, C. Scarparo, V. Penati, D. Nista, S. Bornigia, C. Lacchini, M. Scagnelli, G. Santini, and G. De Sio. 1998. Comparative evaluation of the new Gen-Probe *Mycobacterium tuberculosis* Amplified Direct Test and the semiautomated Abbott LCx *Mycobacterium tuberculosis* Assay for direct detection of *Mycobacterium tuberculosis* Complex in respiratory and extrapulmonary specimens. *J. Clin. Microbiol.* 36:3601–3604.

Reischl, U., N. Lehn, H. Wolf, and L. Naumann. 1998. Clinical evaluation of the automated COBAS AMPLICOR MTB Assay for testing respiratory and nonrespiratory specimens. *J. Clin. Microbiol.* 36:2853–2860.

Ridderhof, J., L. Williams, S. Legois, M. Bussen, B. Metchock, L. Kubista, J. Handsfield, R. Fehd. 1998. Assessment of laboratory performance with nucleic acid amplification (NAA) tests for *Mycobacterium tuberculosis* (*M. tb*). Abstract, Annual Meeting of the American Society for Microbiology.

Riska, P. F., Y. Su, S. Bardarov, L. Freundlich, G. Sarkis, G. Hatfull, C. Carrière, V. Kumar, J. Chan, and W. R. Jacobs, Jr. 1999. Rapid film-based determination of antibiotic suscep-tibilities of *Mycobacterium tuberculosis* strains by using a luciferase reporter phage and the Bronx box. *J. Clin. Microbiol.* 37:1144–1149.

Roberts, G. D., N. L. Goodman, L. Heifets, H. W. Larsh, T. H. Lindner, J. K. McClatchy, M. R. McGinnis, S. H. Siddiqi, and P. Wright. 1983. Evaluation of the BACTEC radiomet-ric method for recovery of mycobacteria and drug susceptibility testing of *Mycobacte-rium tuberculosis* from acid-fast smear-positive specimens. *J. Clin. Microbiol.* 18:689–696.

Rohner, P., E. I. M. Jahn, B. Ninet, C. Ionati, R. Weber, R. Auckenthaler, and G. E. Pfyffer. 1998. Rapid diagnosis of pulmonary tuberculosis with the LCx *Mycobacterium tubercu-losis* Assay and comparison with conventional diagnostic techniques. *J. Clin. Microbiol.* 36:3046–3047.

Royce, S. E. 1999. Personal communication.

Rüsch-Gerdes, S., C. Domehl, G. Nardi, M. R. Gismondo, H.-M. Welscher, and G. E. Pfyffer. 1999. Multicenter evaluation of the Mycobacteria Growth Indicator Tube for testing susceptibility of *Mycobacterium tuberculosis* to first-line drugs. *J. Clin. Microbiol.* 37: 45–48.

Salfinger, M., Y. M. Hale, and J. R. Driscoll. 1998. Diagnostic tools in tuberculosis: present and future. *Respiration* 65:163–170.

Sewell, D. L., and J. D. MacLowry. 1999. Laboratory management, pp. 4–22. *In*: P. R. Murray, E. J. Baron, M. A. Pfaller, F. C. Tenover, and R. H. Yolken (eds.), *Manual of Clinical Microbiology*, 7th ed. ASM Press, Washington, D.C.

Shinnick, T. M., and V. Jonas. 1994. Molecular approaches to the diagnosis of tuberculosis, pp. 517–530. *In*: B. R. Bloom (ed.), *Tuberculosis: Pathogenesis, Protection, and Control*. ASM Press, Washington, D.C.

Skeels, M. 1999. Public health labs in a changing health care landscape. *ASM News* 65:479–483.

Tenover, F. C., J. C. Crawford, R. E. Huebner, L. J. Geiter, C. R. Horsburgh, Jr., and R. C. Good. 1993. The resurgence of tuberculosis: is your laboratory ready? *J. Clin. Microbiol.* 31:767–770.

Tokars, J. I., J. R. Rudnick, K. Kroc, L. Manangan, G. Pugliese, R. E. Huebner, J. Chan, and W. R. Jarvis. 1996. U.S. hospital mycobacteriology laboratories: status and comparison with state public health department laboratories. *J. Clin. Microbiol.* 34:680–685.

van Embden, J. D. A., M. D. Cave, J. T. Crawford, J. W. Dale, K. D. Eisenach, B. Gicquel, P. Hermans, C. Martin, R. McAdam, T. M. Shinnick, and P. M. Small. 1993. Strain identi-fication of *Mycobacterium tuberculosis* by DNA fingerprinting: recommendations for a standardized methodology. *J. Clin. Microbiol.* 31:406–409.

Wang, S. X., and L. Tay. 1999. Evaluation of three nucleic acid amplification methods for direct detection of *Mycobacterium tuberculosis* complex in respiratory specimens. *J. Clin. Microbiol.* 37:1932–1934.

Warren, N. G., and J. R. Cordts. 1996. Activities and recommendations by the Association of State and Territorial Public Health Laboratory Directors. *In*: L. B. Heifits (ed.), *Clinics in Laboratory Medicine: Clinical Mycobacteriology* 16:731–743.

Wobeser, W. L., M. Krajden, J. Conly, H. Simpson, B. Yim, M. D'Costa, M. Fuksa, C. Hiancheong, M. Patterson, A. Phillips, R. Bannatyne, A. Haddad, J. L. Brunton, and S. Krajden. 1996. Evaluation of Roche Amplicor PCR assay for *Mycobacterium tuberculosis*. *J. Clin. Microbiol.* 34:134–139.

Woods, G. I., and F. G. Witebsky. 1993. Current status of mycobacterial testing in clinical laboratories: results of a questionnaire completed by participants in the College of American Pathologists mycobacteriology E survey. *Arch. Pathol. Lab. Med.* 117:876–884.

Yang et al. 1998. Diversity of DNA fingerprints of *Mycobacterium tuberculosis* isolates in the United States. *J. Clin. Microbiol.* 36(4):1003–1007.

Zhou, A. T., W. L. Ma, P. Y. Zhang, and R. A. Cole. 1996. Detection of pulmonary and extrapulmonary tuberculosis patients with the 38-kilodalton antigen from *Mycobacterium tuberculosis* in a rapid membrane-based assay. *Clin. Diagnostic Lab. Immunol.* 3:337–341.

APPENDIX
E

Estimating the Number of Tuberculosis Cases That Can Be Prevented by a Program of Screening and Preventive Therapy of Newly Arrived Immigrants to the United States from Countries with a High Rate of Tuberculosis and the Costs of the Program

The first step in estimating the number of cases that can be prevented by a program of screening and preventive therapy of newly arrived immigrants to the United States from countries with a high rate of tuberculosis was to define the high-risk countries. A recent report on the global burden of tuberculosis included appendixes with a variety of epidemiological measures of tuberculosis burden (Dye et al., 1999). One of the measures was the prevalence of infection for each country. The median prevalence of infection was 36 percent, so any country with a prevalence of infection of >35 percent was defined as a high-tuberculosis-risk country. Fifty-three high-tuberculosis-risk countries were identified, and a list of these countries and their estimated infection prevalences are included in Table E-1.

Mexico had a prevalence of infection estimated at only 17 percent. Although this does not qualify as a high tuberculosis burden on the global scale, it is nearly 2.5 times the rate of infection estimated for the United States. Because of the large number of immigrants to the United States from Mexico, nearly one-quarter of all cases of tuberculosis among the foreign-born in the United States occur among individuals born in Mexico. Therefore, an argument can be made for the inclusion of immigrants from

Mexico in a screening program to identify individuals with latent tuberculosis infection.

The 1996 Statistical Report of the Immigration and Naturalization Service shows that in 1996 421,405 immigrants were admitted to the United States as new arrivals. A total of 187,079 immigrants were admitted from 24 of the high-tuberculosis-risk countries. No immigrants were reported separately in the 1996 statistical report as arriving from the other 29 high-tuberculosis-risk countries, but 4,360 newly arrived immigrants were reported as arriving from other countries in the African, American, Eastern Mediterranean, Southeast Asian, and Western Pacific regions. However, these individuals are not included in further analyses since the precise country of origin could not be ascertained. An additional 52,946 newly arrived immigrants from Mexico were included in the analysis, yielding a total of 240,025 newly arrived immigrants from high-tuberculosis-risk countries and Mexico.

ESTIMATING THE NUMBER OF TUBERCULOSIS CASES

After estimating the number of immigrants to be included in a screening program, the second step is to estimate the number of tuberculosis cases that will occur among these immigrants. Two methods were used to estimate the number of tuberculosis cases. One uses the risk of developing tuberculosis given a positive tuberculin skin test in a population at high risk for infection and with a mixture of old and new infections. The other method uses country- and region-specific annual incidence rates estimated for newly arrived immigrants during the first 5 years in the United States.

The risk of tuberculosis given a positive tuberculin skin test in a population at high risk for infection and with a mixture of old and new infections can be calculated from data for the placebo group of the U.S. Public Health Service trial of isoniazid preventive therapy among household contacts. Patients were enrolled in this trial from 1956 to 1959. Even though nearly 90 percent of these individuals were enrolled as household contacts of individuals with new active cases of tuberculosis, this was very early in the era of tuberculosis chemotherapy (isoniazid was first discovered in 1952) and it is likely that this population had a mixture of recent and old tuberculosis infections. There were 121 cases of tuberculosis among the 4,992 individuals with a tuberculin skin test induration of 10 millimeters or more, for a 5-year risk of tuberculosis in the placebo group of 2.42 percent. By using the individual country estimates of the prevalence of infection and the number of newly arrived immigrants, a total of 87,287 individuals would be infected. With a risk of 2.42 percent, 2,112 cases would be expected to arise in this group in 5 years.

TABLE E-1 Estimated Prevalence of Infection in Countries with an Infection Prevalence of >35% and for Mexico

Region	Country	Infection Prevalence	Region	Country	Infection Prevalence
AFRO	Angola	0.36	EMRO	Djibouti	0.52
	Botswana	0.38		Pakistan	0.4
	Burundi	0.36		Somalia	0.54
	Cape Verde	0.37		Sudan	0.38
	CAR	0.4	EURO		
	Chad	0.4	SEARO	Bangladesh	0.46
	Congo	0.36		Bhutan	0.37
	Democratic Republic of Congo	0.36		Democratic Republic of Korea	0.37
	Equatorial Guinea	0.37		India	0.44
	Eritrea	0.36		Indonesia	0.49
	Ethiopia	0.36		Myanmar (Burma)	0.41
	Gabon	0.37		Nepal	0.45
	Ghana	0.38		Thailand	0.43

	Ivory Coast	0.36	
	Kenya	0.36	
	Liberia	0.37	
	Madagascar	0.37	
	Mauritania	0.36	
	Namibia	0.37	
	Nigeria	0.36	
	South Africa	0.38	
	Swaziland	0.37	
	Togo	0.37	
	Zambia	0.36	
	Zimbabwe	0.36	
AMRO	Bolivia	0.47	
	Equador	0.38	
	Haiti	0.54	
	Peru	0.44	

WPRO	Cambodia	0.64
	People's Republic of China	0.36
	Hong Kong	0.37
	Macau	0.48
	Mongolia	0.45
	New Guinea	0.44
	Philippines	0.47
	Republic of Korea	0.36
	Vietnam	0.44
	Mexico	0.16

TABLE E-2 Summary of Calculation of Estimated Number of
Tuberculosis Cases Among Newly Arrived Immigrants During
the First 5 Years in the United States

World Health Organization Region	Country	No. of Legal Immigrants	Country-Specific 1-Year TB Risk
Africa	Cape Verde	719	0.00176
	Ethiopia	4,622	0.00176
	Ghana	4,387	0.00176
	Kenya	777	0.00176
	Liberia	680	0.00176
	Nigeria	6,426	0.00176
	South Africa	1,309	0.00176
Americas	Bolivia	590	0.00068
	Ecuador	4,816	0.00068
	Haiti	9,189	0.00399
	Peru	5,929	0.00068
Eastern Mediterranean	Pakistan	8,278	0.00113
	Somalia	369	0.00176
	Sudan	805	0.00176
Europe			
Southeast Asia	Bangladesh	6,484	0.00113
	India	30,089	0.00113
	Indonesia	483	0.00113
	Myanmar	1,031	0.00113
Western Pacific	Cambodia	1,047	0.00113
	China	34,512	0.00169
	Hong Kong	5,824	0.00169
	Philippines	39,204	0.00268
	Rep. Korea	9,479	0.00171
	Vietnam	10,030	0.00360
Subtotal		187,079	0
	Mexico	52,946	0.00109
Total		240,025	2,081

No. of Country-Specific Cases During First 5 Years	Infection Prevalence	5-Year TB Risk for Infected Individuals	No. of Cases at 5 years	Mean No. of Cases for the Two Methods
6	0.37	0.0242	6	6
41	0.36	0.0242	40	40
38	0.38	0.0242	40	39
7	0.36	0.0242	7	7
6	0.37	0.0242	6	6
56	0.36	0.0242	56	56
11	0.38	0.0242	12	12
2	0.47	0.0242	7	4
16	0.38	0.0242	44	30
183	0.54	0.0242	120	152
20	0.44	0.0242	63	42
47	0.40	0.0242	80	63
3	0.54	0.0242	5	4
7	0.38	0.0242	7	7
37	0.46	0.0242	72	54
170	0.44	0.0242	320	245
3	0.49	0.0242	6	4
6	0.41	0.0242	10	8
6	0.64	0.0242	16	11
292	0.36	0.0242	301	296
49	0.37	0.0242	52	51
525	0.47	0.0242	446	485
81	0.36	0.0242	83	82
181	0.44	0.0242	107	144
287	0.16	0.0242	205	246
			2,112	2,097

of origin, that cost could be avoided. However, start-up costs for the program were not included in the calculations. Many public health departments will not be prepared for implementation of this kind of program and will incur significant costs in starting up programs for large-scale tuberculin skin testing and treatment of individuals with latent infection. However, it must also be noted that these start-up costs will yield benefits to other programs for tuberculin skin testing and treatment of latent infection that will be needed in the same communities. Costs that would be incurred by the Immigration and Naturalization Service and the Division of Quarantine of the Centers for Disease Control and Prevention to ensure that information on the immigrants is reliably recorded and communicated between Immigration and Naturalization Service and the health department are not included. Costs are also not included for the training and monitoring of the individuals who will perform the tuberculin skin testing for the medical evaluations or for the additional contacts the immigrant that might be required to have with the Immigration and Naturalization Service after evaluation and therapy (if necessary) is completed and the permanent residency card is given out. However, the rapid and reliable flow of information and the training and monitoring should be a requirement for the current program, and many of these costs may be incurred whether screening requirements are changed or not.

TABLE E-3 Costs of Self-Administered Isoniazid-Based Regimen for Treatment of Latent Tuberculosis

Item	Cost	No. of People	Total Cost
Mailings, calls, and visits	See below	242,420	$2,789,563.30
Tuberculin testing	$15.00	236,360	$3,545,392.50
Chest X ray and physician visit	$94.00	86,035	$8,087,276.65
9-month isoniazid therapy	$122.56	68,828	$8,435,545.76
Directly observed therapy			
Laboratory evaluation for adverse reactions	$31.00	69	$2,133.66
Hospital stay for adverse reactions	$5,922	7	$40,759.87
Total cost			$22,900,671.75
No. of cases prevented		1,573	
Cost per case prevented			$14,558.60
Cost per tuberculosis case			$16,391.00

REFERENCES

Catlos et al. 1998. Public health interventions to encourage TB class A/B1/B2 immigrants to present for TB screening. *Am J Respir Crit Care Med* 158(4):1037–1041.

Dye, C., Scheele, S., Dolin, P., Patania, V., et al. 1999. Global burden of tuberculosis: estimated incidence, prevalence, and mortality by country. *JAMA* 282:677–686.

Immigration and Naturalization Service. 1996. 1996 Statistical Report, Table 7, Immigrants admitted by type of admission and region and selected country of birth. Washington, DC: Immigration and Naturalization Service. 1995.

McKenna M, McCray E, Onorato I. The epidemiology of tuberculosis among foreign-born persons in the United States, 1986 to 1993. *N Engl J Med* 332:1071–1076.

Zuber, P., McKenna, M., Binkin, N., Onorato, I., Castro, K. 1997. Long-term risk of tuberculosis among foreign-born persons in the United States. *JAMA* 278:304–307.

APPENDIX
F
Approval Dates for Existing and Prospects for Development of New Antituberculosis Drugs and Vaccines

TABLE F-1 Approval Dates for Antituberculosis Drugs and Vaccines

Drug	FDA Approval Date or Year of First USPHS Published Trial (*)
Isoniazid	1953*
Rifamycins	
rifampin	1974*
rifabutin	12/23/1992
rifapentine	6/22/1998
Pyrazinamide	1959*
Ethambutol	1968*
Streptomycin	1947*
Para-aminosalicylic acid (PAS)	1950*
Ethionamide	1968*
Cycloserine	1968*
Capreomycin	1956*
Kanamycin	Discovered early 1950s; not studied in USPHS trial
Thiacetazone (not available in United States)	—
Fluoroquinolones	
ciprofloxacin	12/26/1990
ofloxacin	12/28/1990
levofloxacin	12/20/1996
Amikacin	Before 1/01/1982

TABLE F-2 Pharmaceutical Companies: Current (1999) Prospects for Development of New Antituberculosis Drugs and Vaccines

Company	New Antimicrobials Available in:			Vaccines
	2 Years	5 Years	8 Years	
Abbott Laboratories	0	0	0	0
American Home Products (Lederle/Wyeth-Ayerst)	0	0	0	0
Astro-Zeneca Pharmaceuticals	0	0	0	0
Bristol-Myers Squibb	0	0	0	0
Dupont Pharmaceuticals	0	?oxazolidinones	?oxazolidinones	0
Eli Lilly and Company	0	0	0	0
Glaxo-Wellcome	0	0	?	Working on vaccines • DNA • Whole attenuated live organism • Therapeutic vaccine
Hoechst Marion Roussel Rifapentine approved by FDA in 1998	0	0	0	0
Janssen Pharmaceuticals	0 0	0 0		
Merck and Company	0 0	0		Very exploratory; have rights to a DNA vaccine in the public domain. Would also be interested in a subunit vaccine

Table continued on next page

246

TABLE F-2 *Continued*

Company	New Antimicrobials Available in:			
	2 Years	5 Years	8 Years	Vaccines
Novartis Pharmaceuticals	0		0	0
Ortho-McNeil Johnson & Johnson	0		Sending some candidate drugs out for in vitro testing; marketing experts not enthusiastic	0
Parke-Davis	0	0	0	0
Pfizer, Inc.	0	0	0	0
Pharmacia/Upjohn	0	?oxazolidinones	?oxazolidinones	0
Rhone-Poulene Rorer	0 0	0 0		
Roche Pharmaceuticals	Had some preliminary work on IL-12 but gave up when in animals it increased CFU in lung	Had some preliminary work on IL-12 but gave up when in animals it increased CFU in lung	Had some preliminary work on IL-12 but gave up when in animals it increased CFU in lung	Had some preliminary work on IL-12 but gave up when in animals it increased CFU in lung
Schering-Plough Corp.	0	0	0	0
G.D. Searle-Monsanto Co.	0	0	0	0
Smith Kline Beecham Pharmaceuticals	0	0	0	0
Warners Chilcott Laboratories	0	0	0	0
Warner Lambert Co.	0	0	0	0

TABLE F-3 Biotechnology Companies: Current (1999) Prospects for Development of New Antituberculosis Drugs and Vaccines

Company	New Antimicrobials Available in:			Vaccines
	2 Years	5 Years	8 Years	
Biogen	0	0	0	0
Corixa Corp.	0	0	0	Vaccines are their approach, not antimicrobials • Collaborating with Smith Kline Beecham • Working on vaccine for 3 years • Have developed a vaccine utilizing 3–5 protein antigens made by incorporating genes for these proteins (a synthetic gene) with effective epitopes (multiple) in one recombinant protein • Efficacy already shown in a rodent model • Safety already shown in monkeys • Clinical trials (Brazil and in another country) phase I/II in approximately 1 year

Table continued on next page

TABLE F-3 Continued

| Company | New Antimicrobials Available in: | | | |
	2 Years	5 Years	8 Years	Vaccines
Genetech	0	0	0	0
Genetics Institute	• IL-12 plus 3 drugs—study vs. TB in Gambia (currently under way) • IL-12 plus 3 drugs—study vs. MA-I in patients with genetic defects in interferon receptor • IL-12 plus 3 drugs—study in treatment of *M. tuberculosis* or MA-I in HIV-infected patients, an ACTG study	?	?	?
Pathogenesis Corp.	• Rifamycin analog (Rifalizyl) with longer half-life cross-resistant with rifampin so not pursuing any longer • PA 824 (a nitroimidizopyrene) under development—active as a drug vs. drug-resistant *M. tuberculosis* (acts by inhibiting glycolipid cell wall synthesis, but at a different step than is inhibited by ethambutol). Presented as a prodrug that is activated in host (as in the case of INH).	0	0	0

1) Activity: mole for mole as active as INH
2) Orally active
3) Bactericidal
4) Active vs. nongrowing organisms (e.g., *M. tuberculosis* cultured under anaerobic conditions)
5) Now in initial stages of testing

Ribozyme Pharmaceuticals	0	0	0
Sequella Corp.	Clinical testing probably	Clinical testing probably	Vaccine: Has license for new experimental vaccine (*Nature* 400[6741]:269; 1999)
	0	0	0

• Ethambutol analogs (3 candidates)
• Shikemic acid pathway (inhibitor)
• New diagnostic being studied: A patch test that may be positive in patients with active disease but not in individuals with prior infection

APPENDIX
G

Committee Biographies

MORTON SWARTZ, M.D. (*Chair*), Harvard Medical School, Massachusetts General Hospital, Boston. Morton Swartz received his M.D. from Harvard Medical School. He is professor of medicine, Harvard Medical School, chief of the James Jackson Firm of the Medical Service, and chief, emeritus, of the Infectious Disease Unit at Massachusetts General Hospital. He is a member of the Institute of Medicine, an associate editor of the *New England Journal of Medicine,* and a master of the American College of Physicians and recipient of its Distinguished Teacher Award. He has served as president of the Infectious Diseases Society of America and has been a recipient of its Bristol Award, as chairman of the Board of Scientific Counselors of the National Institute of Child Health and Human Development, and on the Board of Governors of the American Board of Internal Medicine. His publications cover a variety of clinical and research subjects in the fields of infectious disease and antimicrobial resistance.

RONALD BAYER, Ph.D., Joseph L. Mailman School of Public Health, Columbia University. Ronald Bayer is professor in the Division of Sociomedical Sciences at the Joseph L. Mailman School of Public Health at Columbia University. He received his Ph.D. in political science from the University of Chicago. Since 1982, he has been involved in the study of the ethical and policy dimensions of the AIDS epidemic. He served on the National Research Council's committee to study the social impact of AIDS. He is the author of numerous articles on ethical issues posed by AIDS and tuberculosis and of *Private Acts, Social Consequences: AIDS and the Politics* *of Public Health,* and has edited most recently *Blood Feuds: AIDS, Blood, and the Politics of Medical Disaster.*

C. PATRICK CHAULK, M.D., M.P.H., Annie E. Casey Foundation, Baltimore, Maryland. Patrick Chaulk received his M.D. and completed a residency in pediatrics at the University of Nebraska Medical Center. He also completed a residency and chief residency in preventive medicine at the Johns Hopkins School of Hygiene and Public Health. As the senior associate for health at the Annie Casey Foundation, Dr. Chaulk directs the foundation's investments in health and public health. He also serves as an adjunct faculty member at the Johns Hopkins School of Hygiene and Public Health and the School of Medicine, where he serves as pediatric consultant to Baltimore City's tuberculosis (TB) and sexually transmitted disease (STD) clinics. He has extensive experience in congressional, state, and municipal health and public health public policy regarding TB and STD control. He has written on TB and STD policy and care, public health, and managed care. The recipient of an American Medical Association/ Burroughs-Wellcome Resident Leadership Award, he also was selected as a U.S. Public Health Service Primary Care Health Policy Fellow.

FRAN DU MELLE, M.S., American Lung Association, Washington, D.C. Fran Du Melle is deputy managing director of the American Lung Association. She serves as the director of government relations for the American Lung Association and the American Thoracic Society. She has primary responsibility for the development and implementation of the public policy program, including policy initiatives in environmental health, health care and public health, research advocacy, and tobacco control. Ms. Du Melle's specific areas of expertise include air quality and the public health policy aspects of tuberculosis control and asthma prevention and control.

SUE C. ETKIND, R.N., M.S., Massachusetts Department of Public Health, Boston. Sue Etkind received her diploma in nursing from Concord Hospital School of Nursing and her nursing degree from Fitchburg State College. She graduated from Russell Sage College with a master's degree in health education. She has been the director of the Division of Tuberculosis Prevention and Control since 1984. Ms. Etkind has served on the National Advisory Committee for the Elimination of Tuberculosis, and has been a consultant for the former congressional Office of Technology Assessment, the Centers for Substance Abuse Treatment, and the American Lung Association. She has held positions in the Nursing Section of the International Union Against Tuberculosis and Other Lung Diseases and in its North American region and is the current vice-president of the National

TB Controllers Association. Ms. Etkind was also a recipient of the Lillian Wald Public Service Award presented by the American Public Health Association. She has written extensively on the public health aspects of tuberculosis control.

DAVID FLEMING, M.D., Oregon Health Division, Portland. David Fleming is Oregon's state epidemiologist and oversees Health Division programs in communicable disease prevention; HIV and sexually transmitted diseases; health promotion and chronic disease prevention; environmental, occupational, and injury epidemiology; and vital records and community assessment. He received his M.D. at the State University of New York, his training in internal medicine at Oregon Health Sciences University, and his training in preventive medicine at the Centers for Disease Control and Prevention. He is on the faculty in the Department of Public Health and Preventive Medicine at Oregon Health Sciences University and has authored or coauthored a number of scientific publications. He sits on several national advisory boards and task forces, including the Advisory Committee on Immunization Practices and the U.S. Public Health Service Task Force on Community Preventive Services. He is a past president of CSTE, the national association of state epidemiologists.

AUDREY R. GOTSCH, Dr.P.H., C.H.E.S., University of Medicine and Dentistry of New Jersey (UMDNJ)-School of Public Health. Audrey Gotsch graduated from the University of Michigan School of Public Health (M.P.H.) and the Columbia University School of Public Health (Dr.P.H.). She is professor and interim dean at the UMDNJ School of Public Health. She also serves as director of the Division of Public Education and Risk Communication, Environmental and Occupational Health Sciences Institute, UMDNJ-Robert Wood Johnson Medical School and Rutgers, The State University of New Jersey. Her expertise is in public health, with a specialty in environmental and occupational health education. Dr. Gotsch has been involved in the design, implementation, evaluation, and replication of an environmental and occupational health information program that includes an environmental health sciences curriculum to provide critical thinking skills for youths from kindergarten through 12th grade. She also directs a regional training program that has enhanced the skills of over 180,000 workers in environmental and occupational health content areas. She is the immediate past president of the American Public Health Association, former president of the Council on Education for Public Health, former chair and current member of the New Jersey Public Health Council, and chair of the Board of Directors of the National Center for Health Education.

PHILIP C. HOPEWELL, M.D., San Francisco General Hospital, University of California at San Francisco (UCSF). Dr. Hopewell obtained his M.D. degree from West Virginia University and trained in internal medicine and pulmonary disease at UCSF. Currently, he is professor of medicine at UCSF and associate dean of the School of Medicine. Dr. Hopewell's interest in tuberculosis stems from his time as a medical officer in the U.S. Public Health Service Division of Tuberculosis Control, from which he was assigned to the Pennsylvania Department of Health for 2 years. He has also worked in tuberculosis control programs in Nigeria and Peru. Dr. Hopewell is past president of the American Thoracic Society and the North American region of the International Union Against Tuberculosis and Lung Disease. He was also director of the Robert Wood Johnson Foundation National Tuberculosis Program. Currently, he is medical director of the Francis J. Curry National Tuberculosis Center at UCSF and coordinator of the Tuberculosis Global Action Plan development process, working in collaboration with the World Health Organization. He conducts an active research program in the molecular epidemiology of tuberculosis as well as in other clinical and epidemiological investigative areas.

DONALD R. HOPKINS, M.D., M.P.H., The Carter Center, Chicago. Donald Hopkins is associate executive director of The Carter Center, where he oversees all health programs. He was with the Centers for Disease Control and Prevention for 20 years, the last 3 as deputy director, before moving to The Carter Center in 1987. He is especially interested in disease eradication, having served in the Smallpox Eradication Program. He cochaired the Dahlem Workshop on the Eradication of Infectious Diseases in 1997 and is currently leading the Dracunculiasis (Guinea worm disease) Eradication Program from The Carter Center. He has served on two previous Institute of Medicine committees.

JOHN A. SBARBARO, M.D., M.P.H., University of Colorado Health Sciences Denver, Denver. John Sbarbaro serves as the medical director of University Physicians, Inc., the multispecialty medical group practice of the University of Colorado School of Medicine. A graduate of the Johns Hopkins School of Medicine and the Harvard School of Public Health, he has held professorships in both medicine and preventive medicine since 1983. He has been involved in all aspects of tuberculosis control since 1965 and has been a member of 35 national and international committees or panels and has served as a consultant to the World Health Organization, the Centers for Disease Control and Prevention, the Robert Wood Johnson Foundation, and the U.S. Departments of Health and Human Services and Labor. He has authored 12 book chapters and more than 145 journal publications. He has also served in a variety of leadership roles in the private, public, insurance, and voluntary sectors of medicine.

PETER M. SMALL, M.D., Stanford University Medical Center. Peter Small was trained in internal medicine at the University of California at San Francisco and infectious diseases at Stanford Medical Center. The focus of his research is the nature and consequence of genetic variability within the species *Mycobacterium tuberculosis.* He has published extensively on the use of molecular genotyping in tuberculosis research, particularly as it relates to the evaluation and improvement of tuberculosis control. He has participated actively in research projects in Africa, Asia, Latin America, and Europe. He is currently the director of the Stanford Center for Tuberculosis Research.

MARY E. WILSON, M.D., Harvard Medical School and Harvard School of Public Health, and Mount Auburn Hospital, Cambridge, Mass. Mary E. Wilson graduated from the University of Wisconsin Medical School and is chief of infectious diseases at Mount Auburn Hospital. At Harvard Medical School, she is associate professor of medicine; at Harvard School of Public Health she is associate professor of population and international health. She served on the Advisory Committee for Immunization Practices of the Centers for Disease Control and Prevention from 1988 to 1992 and on the Academic Advisory Committee for the National Institute of Public Health in Mexico. She wrote *A World Guide to Infections: Diseases, Distribution, Diagnosis* (Oxford University Press, 1991) and edited, with R. Levins and A. Spielman, *Disease in Evolution: Global Changes and Emergence of Infectious Diseases* (New York Academy of Sciences, 1994). Her interests include determinants of infectious disease distribution, infections in travelers and immigrants, tuberculosis, and immunizations.

LESTER N. WRIGHT, M.D., M.P.H., New York State Department of Correctional Services, Albany. Lester N. Wright is associate commissioner and chief medical officer responsible for provision of health care to 72,000 inmates in New York State prisons. He is certified by the American Board of Preventive Medicine. He has served as county and state health director (commissioner). He spent 7 years working in various parts of Africa in the delivery of primary health care and health system development and supervision. He continues to do international consultation in areas such as child survival and HIV prevention. He has dealt with tuberculosis in primary care in Ethiopia, and has been a TB control officer for a county public health agency and a state health officer. During his term at the Department of Correctional Services, multiple drug-resistant TB was first identified among prisoners and new cases of TB have decreased 83 percent since their peak in 1991.

Liaison from the Board on International Health

BARRY R. BLOOM, Ph.D., dean of the Harvard School of Public Health and professor of immunology and infectious disease. Barry R. Bloom received his B.A. and an honorary Sc.D. from Amherst College and his Ph.D. from the Rockefeller University. Dr. Bloom is an immunologist and microbiologist engaged in research on infectious diseases and vaccines. Before going to Harvard, Dr. Bloom was an investigator of the Howard Hughes Medical Institute and the Weinstock Professor of Microbiology and Immunology at the Albert Einstein College of Medicine. He is a member of the Scientific Advisory Board of the National Center for Infectious Diseases at the Centers for Disease Control and Prevention. He chairs the Board of Trustees of the newly established International Vaccine Institute and is cochair of the Board on Global Health of the Institute of Medicine. He is chairman of the Vaccine Advisory Committee of UNAIDS and a member of the U.S. AIDS Vaccine Research Committee. In 1991, he received the first Bristol-Myers Squibb Award for Distinguished Research in Infectious Diseases and in 1998 received the Novartis Prize in Immunology. Dr. Bloom is a member of the National Academy of Sciences, the American Academy of Arts and Sciences, and the Institute of Medicine.

Liaison to the Board on Health Promotion and Disease Prevention

ROBERT FULLILOVE, Ed.D., Columbia University School of Public Health. Robert Fullilove received his Ed.D. from Columbia University. He is currently the associate dean for community and minority affairs at Columbia University's School of Public Health. He is also an associate professor of clinical public health and the codirector of the Community Research Group at the New York State Psychiatric Institute. His research includes HIV disease among people of color, crack cocaine use and sexually transmitted disease in the AIDS era, and trauma-related disorders and their impact on sexual risk taking. He is a member of the Board of Health Promotion and Disease Prevention of the Institute of Medicine and has served as a member/nominee to the Centers for Disease Control and Prevention's Advisory Committee on HIV and STD Prevention.

Index